Professional Practical/Vocational Nursing

Professional Practical/Vocational Nursing

LOIS HARRION, MS, RN
Nurse Consultant
L'MARCA Consulting & Associates

Director of Vocational Nursing
Simi Valley Adult School
Simi Valley, CA

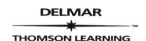

DELMAR
™
THOMSON LEARNING

Australia Canada Mexico Singapore Spain United Kingdom United States

NOTICE TO THE READER

Publisher does not warrant or guarantee any of the products described herein or perform any independent analysis in connection with any of the product information contained herein. Publisher does not assume, and expressly disclaims, any obligation to obtain and include information other than that provided to it by the manufacturer.

The reader is expressly warned to consider and adopt all safety precautions that might be indicated by the activities herein and to avoid all potential hazards. By following the instructions contained herein, the reader willingly assumes all risks in connection with such instructions.

The Publisher makes no representation or warranties of any kind, including but not limited to, the warranties of fitness for particular purpose or merchantability, nor are any such representations implied with respect to the material set forth herein, and the publisher takes no responsibility with respect to such material. The publisher shall not be liable for any special, consequential, or exemplary damages resulting, in whole or part, from the readers' use of, or reliance upon, this material.

Delmar Staff:

Business Unit Director: William Brottmiller
Acquisitions Editor: Matthew Filimonov
Editorial Assistant: Melissa A. Longo
Executive Marketing Manager: Dawn Gerrain

Channel Manager: Tara Carter
Project Editor: Mary Ellen Cox
Production Coordinator: Anne Sherman
Art/Design Coordinator: Timothy J. Conners

COPYRIGHT © 2001 Delmar, a division of Thomson Learning, Inc. Thomson Learning™ is a trademark used herein under license.

Printed in Canada
1 2 3 4 5 6 7 8 9 10 XXX 05 04 03 02 01 00

For more information, contact Delmar, 3 Columbia Circle, PO Box 15015, Albany, NY 12212-0515; or find us on the World Wide Web at http://www.delmar.com

ASIA (including India):
Thomson Learning
60 Albert Street, #15-01
Albert Complex
Singapore 189969
Tel 65 336-6411
Fax 65 336-7411

AUSTRALIA/NEW ZEALAND:
Nelson
102 Dodds Street
South Melbourne
Victoria 3205
Australia
Tel 61 (0)3 9685-4111
Fax 61 (0)3 9685-4199

LATIN AMERICA:
Thomson Learning
Seneca 53
Colonia Polanco
11560 Mexico, D.F. Mexico
Tel (525) 281-2906
Fax (525) 281-2656

CANADA:
Nelson
1120 Birchmount Road
Toronto, Ontario
Canada M1K 5G4
Tel (416) 752-9100
Fax (416) 752-8102

UK/EUROPE/MIDDLE EAST/AFRICA:
Thomson Learning
Berkshire House
168-173 High Holborn
London WC1V 7AA
United Kingdom
Tel 44 (0)20 497-1422
Fax 44 (0)20 497-1426

Business Press
Berkshire House
168-173 High Holborn
London WC1V 7AA
United Kingdom
Tel 44 (0)20 497-1422
Fax 44 (0)20 497-1426

SPAIN (includes Portugal):
Paraninfo
Calle Magallanes 25
28015 Madrid
Espana
Tel 34 (0)91 446-3350
Fax 34 (0)91 445-6218

DISTRIBUTION SERVICES:
ITPS
Cheriton House
North Way
Andover,
Hampshire SP10 5BE
United Kingdom
Tel 44 (0)1264 34-2960
Fax 44 (0)1264 34-2759

INTERNATIONAL HEADQUARTERS:
Thomson Learning
International Division
290 Harbor Drive, 2nd Floor
Stamford, CT 06902-7477
Tel (203) 969-8700
Fax (203) 969-8751

FOREIGN RIGHTS DEPARTMENT (Headquarters:)
Thomson Learning
Berkshire House
168-173 High Holborn
London WC1V 7AA
United Kingdom
Tel 44 (0)20 497-1422
Fax 44 (0)20 497-1426

FOREIGN RIGHTS—ASIA:
Thomson Learning
60 Albert Street, #15-01
Albert Complex
Singapore 189969
Tel 65 336-6411
Fax 65 334-1617

FOREIGN RIGHTS—SPAIN:
Paraninfo
Calle Magallanes 25
28015 Madrid
Espana
Tel 34 (0)91 446-3350
Fax 34 (0)91 445-6218

FOREIGN RIGHTS—LATIN AMERICA:
Thomson Learning
Seneca 53
Colonia Polanco
11560 Mexico, D.F. Mexico
Tel (525) 281-2906
Fax (525) 281-2656

Library of Congress Cataloging-in-Publication Data

Harrion, Lois.
    Professional practical/vocational nursing / Lois Harrion.
        p. cm.
    Includes bibliographical references
    ISBN 0-7668-2275-3
    1. Practical nursing. 2. Nursing—Study and teaching. I. Title.
RT62 .H333 2001
610.73'06'93—dc21   00-052285

Contents

➡ **CHAPTER 5: Ethical Nursing Practice**   157

> **CHAPTER 6: Critical Thinking in Nursing Practice**   **185**

Preface

Professional Practical/Vocational Nursing evolved out of my experiences with nursing students in the final phase of their basic nursing program as well as their transition into nursing practice. This work represents a conscientious effort to present in a stimulating and engaging format, content that will assist graduating students in their careers as nurses.

Nurses today need to know and understand the social and regulatory environment within which they operate. New nurses need to think critically and make the necessary adjustments to changes. The rapidly progressing body of nursing knowledge, the phenomenal technological advances reshaping nursing care, and the colossal changes occurring in the health care delivery system demand more and more from nurses. Each chapter was therefore developed with the changes in the health care delivery system in mind.

Although all nurses—regardless of education or experience—will benefit from a review of *Professional Practical/Vocational Nursing*, the book is primarily intended for practical/vocational nursing programs. Typically, students in the final phase of their education will take a course discussing many of the professional issues contained within this book. Very often it is called "Professional Vocational Relations" or "Professional Management."

Professional Practical/Vocational Nursing provides an overview of the nursing profession from past historical events to the present day. Legal, ethical, and on-the-job issues that today's nurse must be aware of are discussed in light of nursing's evolution. Workplace tips are also provided. Communication in the workplace, how to write an effective résumé, and interviewing tips are among the sound career advancement tools included.

There are also several features included within *Professional Practical/ Vocational Nursing* that are designed to enhance student learning. Each chapter begins with a set of objectives to guide the learning experience followed by a list of key terms that will be used throughout that particular chapter. Additionally, each chapter is summarized with key points, and critical thinking activities provide students with the opportunity to apply the content of the chapter to typical situations encountered in the health care environment.

In addition to the learning objectives and references characteristic in textbooks of this nature, this book has some very creative case studies that are designed to promote critical thinking. Other important features include: a discussion of the various types of institutions and agencies that provide care, from the traditional acute-care hospitals to community-based clinics; the financing of health care, including government-supported and managed care programs; the evolution of nursing as a profession, including nursing traditions and trends; educational preparation for practical/vocational nursing, legal and ethical accountabilities; chapters on critical thinking, leadership and management, and a chapter on transcultural nursing; and Internet resources are provided for each chapter. Ask Yourself boxes are included within each chapter, which provide the student with an opportunity to deal with self-reflection and opinions on various topics. This feature helps the student develop sensitivity and heighten awareness to various issues, and assists with critical thinking and problem solving.

Finally, appendices provide resources that are valuable to the graduate after the basic practical/vocational nursing curriculum is completed. The author recognizes the nursing student as an active participant who assumes a collaborative role in the learning process.

Acknowledgments

This textbook is the product of many conscientious and dedicated people. First, I would like to thank all the reviewers who critically read and commented on the manuscript. Your academic expertise provided valuable suggestions that strengthened the text.

At the risk of being saccharine, I cannot adequately express the depth of my feelings concerning the special contribution of my husband, Milton. He performed technological feats above the call of duty, and more importantly, he permitted me the time and the freedom to fulfill a commitment that I wished to assume.

Special thanks to Ms. Patti Burhans whose technical support was immeasurable. My sincerest thanks to Matt Filimonov, acquisitions editor, who provided support, resources, knowledge, and guidance to make this manuscript a reality. And, he did this with cheer and care.

List of Reviewers

Carol Nelson, RN, MSN
Spokane Community College

Jean Nix, RNC, MSN, MA, PhD
Glendale Community College

Elizabeth Schaeffer Teichler, PhD, RNC, FNP, HNC
CUHSC School of Nursing

Esther Gonzales, RN, MSN, MSEd
Del Mar College

Lou Ann Boose, RN, BSN, MSN
Harrisburg Area Community College

Gail J. Smith, RN, MSN
Miami Dade Community College

Kathy White, RN
Sikeston Public School
Practical Nurse Program

Suellen S. Klein, RN, MSN
Lake Michigan College

Dedication

This text is dedicated to my *students*, who throughout the years have enhanced my journey. And especially to my daughter, Karma, who continuously shows me how to *live* every day of my life.

CHAPTER 1

The Evolution of Nursing

CHAPTER OVERVIEW

This chapter provides an introduction to nursing as a whole. It includes a brief history of nursing as well as definitions of nursing formulated by nursing leaders and nursing organizations. Educational preparation, professional organizations, and guidelines for nursing practice serve as a basis for understanding what nursing is and how it is organized. Finally, because nursing is a part of an ever-changing society, a brief discussion of current trends in nursing is also included.

OBJECTIVES

Upon completion of this chapter, the reader should be able to:

- Describe the evolution of nursing and nursing education from early civilization to the twentieth century.
- List the major developments of practical/vocational nursing.
- Discuss six people important to the development of nursing.
- Describe the purpose, role, and responsibilities of the practical/vocational nurse.
- Discuss the Standards of Practice as described by the American Nurses Association and the Canadian Nurses Association.
- Define the purposes of nursing professional organizations.
- Describe expanded career roles and functions of nurses.
- Describe the three categories of nursing actions.

INTRODUCTION

Nursing is difficult to describe clearly or to define. When the question is asked, many different responses are given. Each person provides an answer based on his or her own personal experience and knowledge of nursing at that time. As you progress toward graduation and as you practice nursing after graduation, those definitions will change, reflecting changes within yourself as you learn about and experience nursing.

Most basically defined, nursing is the care of others. That care involves any number of activities, ranging from carrying out complicated technical procedures to something as seemingly simple as holding a hand. All nursing actions focus on the person receiving care and are a blend of both the art and the science of nursing. The science of nursing is the underlying knowledge base for patient care. The art of nursing is the more personal application of that knowledge to help others reach maximum function and quality of life.

A HISTORICAL BACKGROUND

Nursing evolved over many years, influenced by attitudes toward the sick and the methods available. Changes in the way people live, the interrelationship of people with their environments, the search for knowledge and truth, and technological advances have all made nursing and nursing education both what they are and what they will be. Nursing evolves as society and health care needs and policies change. Nursing responds and adapts to these changes, meeting new challenges as they arise.

The Early Civilizations

From the beginning of time, the nurse has been regarded as a caregiver. This role has traditionally been defined by the groups, communities, and societies in which nursing was practiced. Health care and nursing as we currently know them are based on what has happened in the past.

In 5000 BC there were few references to nursing. **Illness**, an abnormal process in which aspects of the social, emotional, or intellectual condition and function of a person are diminished or impaired, was considered to be directly related to disfavor with God. Early peoples believed that a person became sick when an evil spirit entered the body, and that the presence of a good spirit kept disease away.

In early civilizations, people believed that illness had supernatural causes. The theory of animism was developed in an attempt to understand the cause of the mysterious changes in bodily functions. This theory was based on the belief that everything was alive with invisible forces and endowed with power. Good spirits brought health; evil spirits brought sickness and death. The roles of the physician and the nurse were separate and distinct.

Medicine men performed witchcraft on the affected part of the body to induce the bad spirits to leave the body. Some of the techniques involved the use of frightening masks, noises, incantations, vile odors, charms, spells, and even sacrifices. The physician was the medicine man, and other modes of treatment included chanting, inspiring fear, or opening the skull to release evil spirits. Men assisted the medicine men in treating illnesses. They used purgatives, emetics, application of hot and cold substances, cauterization, cupping, blistering, and massage. Few women assisted the medicine men; women most assisted in childbirth. The nurse usually was the mother who cared for her family during sickness by providing physical care and herbal remedies. This nurturing and caring role of the nurse has continued to the present.

The Babylonians were intellectually, socially, and scientifically well developed. Many wars brought misery, suffering, illness, and injury to their people. There is evidence that some form of medical service existed and that laypersons provided this service. It is believed that these caregivers were usually men. If they were women, they were probably of low status because the actions of Babylonian women were dominated by men.

The ancient Hebrews, according to the Talmud and the Old Testament, attributed their misfortunes and illnesses to God's wrath. They depended on Him to restore them to **health**, a condition of physical, mental, and social well-being and the absence of disease or other abnormal conditions, when they were sick. They combined their religious beliefs with the hygienic practices that were required from Babylon, where they had been in captivity. These practices included the inspection of all meats and the careful selection and preparation of all foods. They prevented the spread of communicable disease by burning infected garments and scrubbing the home of those infected with the disease. Nurses were mentioned occasionally in the Talmud as persons caring for the sick in their homes. This appears to have been a demonstration of the first public health/home care movement. Ancient records of early Egyptian civilization describe nursing procedures, such as feeding a patient, a recipient of a health care service, with tetanus and dressing wounds.

Records of pre-Christian India detail the establishment of hospitals where the sick were cared for. The report described a body of attendants, probably male, who were of good behavior, who were distinguished for purity and cleanliness of habits, and who were clever, skillful, and endowed with kindness. They bathed patients, made beds, and were always willing to do whatever they could to assist the sick.

Hellenic Civilization

By 500 BC the Hellenic civilization showed keen intellect, independent thinking, democratic action, and a thirst for knowledge and truth. Medicine, the art and science of the diagnosis, treatment, and prevention of disease and the maintenance of good health, progressed from the belief that demons and spirits caused human ills to the founding of temples suitable for rest and restoration of health. These temples, often referred to as hospitals, resembled our health centers of today; they had spas, mineral springs, bath gymnasiums, and treatment and consultation rooms. The religious influence was still present in the form of prayer, thanks offerings, and rituals. Priestesses served as attendants and cared for the sick. Pregnant women and people with incurable diseases were not admitted.

Hippocrates, born in 460 BC on the island of Cos in the Mediterranean, was a brilliant, progressive physician and teacher. He rejected the belief in the supernatural origin of disease and adopted a system of physical assessment, observation, and record keeping as an integral part of patient care. As his patient-centered care approach and medical ethics were adopted, Hippocrates was named the "Father of Medicine" and is credited with the Hippocratic oath, which is still taken by physicians today. The work of Hippocrates is the basis for the **holistic**, of or pertaining to the whole; considering all factors, as holistic medicine, approach to patient care.

The Greek influence on the care of the sick changed the approach from one of mysticism to that of public health and safety. Religious influence was still prevalent but with an emphasis on the poor, the sick, the widowed, and the children.

The Christian Influence

With the beginning of Christianity, nursing began to have a formal and more clearly defined role. Led by the belief that love and caring for others were important, women called deaconesses made the first organized visits to sick people, and members of male religious orders gave nursing care and buried the dead. Both male and female nursing orders were founded during the Crusades.

Deacons and deaconesses were designated by the Roman bishops to assist the church by providing services such as visiting sick women in their homes and watching over the sick in the hospitals. One of the first deaconesses, Phoebe, performed nursing functions about AD 60. She was known as a visiting nurse, attending the sick and poor in their homes. Another Roman woman, Fabiola, spent her wealth and time nursing the sick and poor. She is credited with providing the first free hospital in Rome in AD 390.

Monastic and military orders were charged with caring for the sick over the next 1,000 years, but the decline of Roman civilization hindered the progress made in Greece and Rome. Famine, disease, war, and the emphasis on survival resulted in an increased need to care for the sick and poor, but the ongoing battles between the church and state hindered the development of any one approach to patient care. Care of the sick was performed by both men and women. Female religious orders were concerned with the care of the sick and needy, but the concern for religious problems took priority. Male military personnel served the medical needs of soldiers on the battlefield.

At the beginning of the sixteenth century, society changed from one with a religious orientation to one that emphasized warfare, exploration, and expansion of knowledge. Many monasteries and convents closed, leading to a tremendous shortage of people to care for the sick. To meet this need, women who had committed crimes were recruited into nursing in lieu of serving jail sentences. Along with a poor reputation, nurses received low pay and worked long hours in unfavorable conditions.

The Nineteenth Century

In the early nineteenth century, hospitals were overcrowded, and there was a lack of trained and qualified people who were interested in caring for the sick and the infirm. Hospitals were a place to contract diseases rather than be cured of them because of patients with open wounds and unchecked infection and the dirty physical conditions of the hospital. Women of "proper upbringing" did not work outside of the home during this time. As a result, nursing attracted those with fewer opportunities—most often women with little or no education who were reputed to drink heavily and engage in prostitution. The best sources of nurses were the religious nursing orders, but these orders could not begin to meet the ever-increasing need for nursing services. From the middle of the eighteenth century to the nineteenth century, social reforms changed the role of nurses and of women in general.

The Lutheran Order of Deaconesses established the first real school of nursing under the guidance of Theodor Fliedner, a German pastor in Kaiserwerth, Germany. The reputation of the school spread throughout Europe. It reached a young woman in England whose interest in nursing overshadowed the opposition of her family, her friends, and the social class to which she belonged. Florence Nightingale was born in 1820 to a wealthy family. She grew up in England and was well educated and traveled extensively. Despite strong opposition from her family, Nightingale, a strong-minded, intelligent, and determined young woman joined the Kaiserwerth program in 1851 at the age of 31.

Armed with the education and training she received at Kaiserwerth and with her administrative and organizational skills, Florence Nightingale became the superintendent of a charity hospital for ill governesses in 1852. The governing board of the hospital was not always pleased with the changes and innovations she made and the guidance she gave her uneducated nurses, even though the quality of patient care improved.

In the following year, when she was to become superintendent of King's College Hospital in London, news of the atrocious conditions befalling the wounded soldiers in the Crimean War reached England. People were greatly concerned over the number of casualties and deaths that were reported. The outbreak of the Crimean War and a request by the British to organize nursing care for a military hospital in Turkey gave Nightingale an opportunity for achievement. Figure 1–1 shows Florence Nightingale caring for patients in the Crimea.

The secretary of war, a long-standing friend of Miss Nightingale's, asked her to lead a group of nurses to Scutari, Turkey, to care for the wounded. Ironically, she had sent him a letter offering her services at about the same time. Within a week of receiving the secretary's letter, she and thirty-eight nurses left England for Turkey.

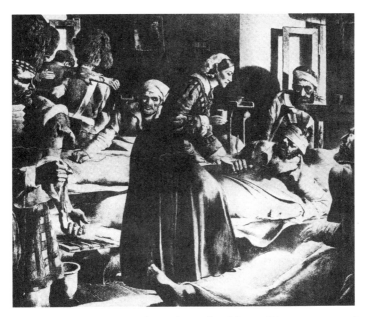

FIGURE 1–1 Florence Nightingale in the Crimea *(Photo courtesy of Parke-Davis & Company, a subsidiary of Warner-Lambert Company)*

Once again Florence Nightingale applied the principles of nursing she had learned at Kaiserwerth. These concepts, coupled with her dedication and leadership, turned the tide. The hospital units were cleaned, clothes were washed regularly, and sanitary conditions, which had been nonexistent, were established. The mortality among the casualties dropped significantly. Not only had the physical environment of the hospital been changed by Florence Nightingale's actions, but through her patience, dedication, and empathetic treatment of the soldiers, a psychological change took place as well. The soldiers grew to respect her and looked forward to her presence on the wards. They looked for her smile and took strength from her self-fulfilled personality. When she made her rounds through the wards late at night, she carried a lamp to light her way through the rows of beds of the injured and sick. This practice became a ritual, and soon she was known as "The Lady with the Lamp." The small lamp she carried became her trademark and continues to be the symbol of the nursing profession around the world.

Because she was able to overcome enormous difficulties successfully, Nightingale challenged prejudices against women and elevated the status of all nurses. After the war, she returned to England, where she established a training school for nurses and wrote books about health care and nursing education.

In 1860 Florence Nightingale began the reformation of nursing from occupation to profession by establishing a nursing school at Saint Thomas Hospital in London. She chose this hospital for the location of the school because of its reputation as a progressive medical facility. It was therefore an ideal place to promote the new standards of nursing that she so strongly believed in.

The nursing program operated separately from the hospital and was financially independent to ensure that the major emphasis of its activity was directed exclusively toward educating nursing students. A nurses' residence was provided for the students, who had to pass strict admission procedures. The length of nurses' education was one year and included both formal instruction and practical experience. Complete records were kept on each student's progress while at the school. This practice became known as the "Nightingale Plan," which was to become the model for nursing education in the twentieth century. After the students graduated, records were also kept on where they were employed. This eventually became a "register," which was the beginning of a movement to exercise control over the nursing graduate and to establish a standard for the practicing nurse.

Students admitted into the nursing program at Saint Thomas had to provide excellent character references, showing a strong commitment to a career in nursing, and had to demonstrate that they were intellectually capable of passing the course of study before them. The resultant demand for "Nightingale nurses" was overwhelming. The improved patient care provided by this new breed of nurses included such measures as good hygiene, sanitation, patient observation, accurate record keeping, nutritional improvements, and the introduction and use of certain new medical equipment.

 ASK YOURSELF

Florence Nightingale as a Model

Florence Nightingale is often thought of as being strong minded and assertive. Why are these important characteristics of nurses? How could these traits be cultivated in nurses today?

The standards of nursing care established by Florence Nightingale gained the respect of the medical community and led to improved care for the sick and a much improved image of nursing in general. The need for educated and trained nurses became painfully evident, and the time was right for a shift in the approach to nursing education.

North America in the Nineteenth Century

During the time Florence Nightingale was active in Europe, the same kinds of patient care problems were occurring in America. The Civil War was characterized by severe casualties, disease, infected wounds, and archaic medical care. As in the Crimean War, nurses were scarce and those who were available were poorly trained to handle the horrors of war. Women such as Dorothea Dix, superintendent of Female Nurses of the Union Army in 1861, and Clara Barton, the founder of the Red Cross in 1881, tried to meet the needs of both the battlefield casualties and civilian casualties. Figure 1–2 pictures women who cared for soldiers during the Civil War.

By the end of the nineteenth century, three schools of nursing were established in the United States. In May 1873 the Bellevue Hospital School of Nursing in New York established itself as the foremost proponent of the Nightingale Plan in America. In October of that same year the Connecticut Training School was opened in New Haven. In November the Boston Training School at the Massachusetts General Hospital began operating. All three were modeled after the Nightingale Plan.

In the interest of establishing standards for the new nursing schools, dedicated women such as Isabelle Hampton Robb and Lavinia Dock organized the American Society of Superintendents of Training Schools of Nursing in 1894. The major goal of this organization was to set educational standards for nurses. The structure of the organization was modeled after that of the American Medical Association. A code of ethics for nurses was adopted by the Society, and this code, known as the Nightingale Pledge, is subscribed to by the nursing profession of today.

The work of Florence Nightingale and the care for Civil War battle casualties demonstrated the need for educated nurses in both Canada and the United States. The first schools of nursing were founded—usually in connection with hospitals. Although these schools were established on the beliefs of Nightingale, the training they provided was based more on apprenticeship than on educational programs. Hospitals saw an economic advantage in having their own school. Most hospital schools were organized to provide a ready source of

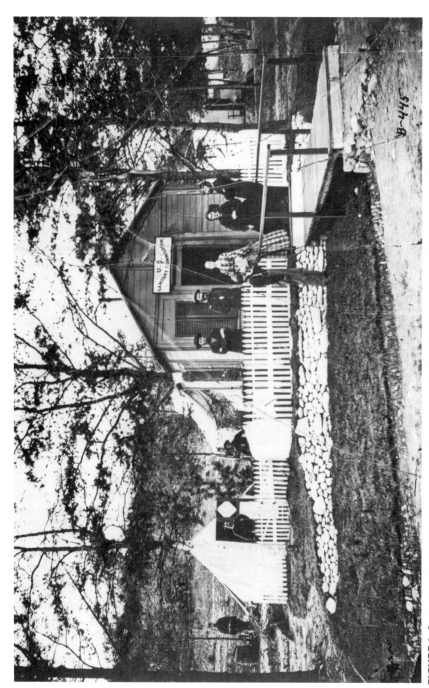

FIGURE 1–2 During the Civil War, women were instrumental in the effort to minimize the risk of spreading contagious diseases among wounded soldiers. *(Photo courtesy of Corbis-Bettman)*

easily controlled and inexpensive staff. This resulted in the loss of clear guidelines separating nursing service and nursing education. As students and as graduates, female nurses were under the control of male hospital administrators and physicians. The lack of educational standards, the male dominance of health care, and the pervading Victorian belief that women depended on men combined to contribute to several decades of slow progress toward professionalism in nursing.

Florence Nightingale's Legacy

Despite these negative circumstances, Florence Nightingale's contributions are undeniable. They are numerous and far-reaching.

- Identifying personal needs of the patient and the role of the nurse in meeting those needs
- Establishing standards for hospital management
- Establishing a respected occupation for women
- Establishing nursing education
- Recognizing the two components of nursing—health and illness
- Believing that nursing is separate and distinct from medicine
- Recognizing that nutrition is important to health
- Instituting occupational and recreational therapy for sick people
- Stressing the need for continuing education for nurses
- Maintaining accurate records that are recognized as the beginnings of nursing research

Florence Nightingale elevated the status of nursing to a respected occupation, improved the quality of nursing care, and founded modern nursing education. Table 1–1 lists persons who were important to the development of nursing.

 ASK YOURSELF

Characteristics of Nursing Leaders

Personal influence comes to those who are clear about their goals and who view their work as essential to reaching those goals. As you read about nursing leaders, consider the traits that enabled them to shape nursing's future in health care.

TABLE 1–1

People Important to the Development of Nursing in the Nineteenth and Early Twentieth Centuries

Person	Contribution
Clara Barton	Volunteered to care for wounds and feed soldiers during the Civil War; served as the supervisor of nurses for the Army of James, organizing hospitals and nurses; established the Red Cross in the United States in 1882.
Dorothea Dix	Superintendent of the Female Nurses of the Army during the Civil War; was given the authority and the responsibility for recruiting and equipping a corps of army nurses; was a pioneering crusader for the reform of the treatment of the mentally ill.
Mary Ann Bickerdyke	Organized diet kitchens, laundries, an ambulance service, and supervised nursing staff during the Civil War.
Louise Schuler	A nurse during the Civil War, she returned to New York and organized the New York Charities Aid Association; this organization worked to improve care of the sick in Bellevue Hospital; one recommendation was to have standards for nursing education.
Linda Richards	The first trained nurse in the United States; a graduate of the New England Hospital for Women and Children in Boston, Massachusetts in 1873; became the night superintendent of Bellevue Hospital in 1874 and began the practice of keeping records and writing orders.
Jane Addams	Provided social services within a neighborhood setting; a leader for women's rights; recipient of the 1931 Nobel Peace Prize.
Lillian Wald	Established a neighborhood nursing service for the sick poor of the lower East Side of New York City; founder of public health nursing.
Mary Elizabeth Mahoney	Graduated from the New England Hospital for Women and Children in 1879 as America's first black nurse.

Table 1–1 *continued*

Harriet Tubman	A nurse and an abolitionist, she was active in the underground railroad movement before joining the Union Army during the Civil War.
Nora Gertrude Livingston	Established a training program for nurses at the Montreal General Hospital (the first three-year program in North America).
Mary Agnes Sniverly	Director of the school at Toronto General Hospital and one of the founders of the Canadian Nurses Association.
Sojourner Truth	A nurse who not only provided care to the soldiers during the Civil War, but also worked for the women's movement.
Isabel Hampton Robb	A leader in nursing and nursing education, she organized the nursing school at Johns Hopkins Hospital, where she initiated policies that included limiting the number of hours in a day's work; wrote a textbook to help student learning; was the first president of the Nurses Associated Alumnae of the United States and Canada (which later became the American Nurses Association).
Florence Nightingale	A nursing leader considered to be the founder of modern nursing; established the Nightingale Training School of Nurses at St. Thomas Hospital in London; revolutionized the method for educating nurses; advocated a systematic method of assessing patients, individualized care, and maintaining confidentiality.
Mary Adelaide Nutting	As a member of the faculty of Teachers' College, Columbia University, she became the first professor of nursing in the world and, with Livinia Dock, published the four-volume *History of Nursing*.
Elizabeth Smellie	A member of the original Victoria Order of Nurses for Canada (a group that provided public health nursing); organized the Canadian Women's Army Corps during World War II.
Lavinia Dock	A nursing leader and women's rights activist who was instrumental in the constitutional amendment giving women the right to vote.
Mary Beckenridge	Established the Frontier Nursing Service and one of the first midwifery schools in the United States.

Florence Nightingale left a legacy of roles and lessons that are as applicable today as they were a hundred years ago.

The Innovator

Stand up for your beliefs. Innovate. Create systems so people can do their jobs effectively and efficiently.

The Manager

Let your boss know what has been accomplished. Establish standards. Use hospitals only when necessary.

The Statistician

The systematic approach of outcomes is critical. A graph is an effective communication tool. In order to compare results, you must have standardized data.

The Patient Care Administrator

Always be prepared for the unexpected. Patience is more effective than aggression. Timing is everything. Create effective systems for obtaining and distributing resources. Caring for the sick requires a holistic approach.

The Nurse

Providing comfort and caring helps the patient and rewards the caregiver. A healthy environment is essential to good patient care. You don't have to do everything yourself, but you do have to make sure everything gets done.

The Reformer

Enlist competent people. Learn to translate your message for a variety of audiences. Know who has the power and what they value. Persist!

The Collaborator

Be realistic. The best way to influence results is often to do the behind-the-scenes work. Know your audience.

The Educator

Health care education should be a multidisciplined effort. Detailed feedback is essential to performance improvement. Performance evaluation is a two-way street. Networking is a key to organizational and personal success.

The Architect

Design health care facilities that meet the needs of the patients and the staff.

The Communicator

Communicate, communicate, communicate!

The Time Manager

Plan uninterrupted time to think.

The Twentieth Century

While the superintendents of the nurses' training schools organized at the national level, the graduates of those training schools organized in their own fashion at local levels. They established the Alumnae Association in an attempt to establish standards for the actual practice of nursing.

Changes in nursing education and practice did not occur in a vacuum. Any change was affected by the social issues of the times. The late nineteenth and early twentieth centuries were a time of growing legislation and standardization. People were trying to improve their world by regulating both personal and organizational behavior. This desire saw its expression in movements such as temperance laws and antitrust legislation. It is not surprising that this tendency would also make an impact in nursing education.

In 1903 the first nursing licensure laws to protect the public were passed in North Carolina, New Jersey, New York, and Virginia. These laws required that a governing body grant an individual permission to engage in an activity that would otherwise be illegal. As a result, the nursing organizations recognized the need to amend their purpose and redirect their focus. As part of the reorganization that followed, the American Society of Superintendents of Training Schools became the Education Committee of the National League for Nursing Education in 1903. The Alumnae Association became the American Nurses Association in 1911.

Concurrent with these changes, Isabelle Hampton Robb (Figure 1–3) and Mary Adelaide Nutting developed a program at Columbia University to train and develop teachers of nursing. They were convinced that nurses needed not only a college education and clinical practice, but also specific training in theoretical knowledge. The belief that nurses needed such a balance of liberal arts education and nursing practice skills brought a new perspective to the profession of nursing.

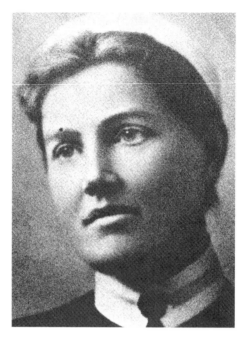

FIGURE 1–3 Isabel Hampton Robb *(Photo courtesy of the American Nurses Association)*

World War I brought an increased demand for nurses. The newly formed Army and Navy Nurse Corps sought nurses who school super-intendents certified as having "good moral character and professional qualifications." The available supply of nurses could not meet the demand, so once again untrained women volunteered their services to their country. Nursing leaders, concerned that these untrained person-nel would be caring directly for wounded and ailing soldiers without adequate training, quickly established the Army School of Nursing.

World War I escalated the need for trained nurses abroad, while in the United States, the Spanish influenza epidemic strained the resources of the nursing community. The Smith-Hughes Act was passed in 1917 to provide vocational and public education. Federal funding then provided the means for vocational-based practical/vocational nursing programs throughout the country. Even with these resources, the demand for nurses caused by war and epidemic could not be met.

After the war the women who served as military nurses returned to their homes and their previous jobs and careers. They had no desire to remain in nursing as civilians. The image attached to professional nurses still posed a problem for most women. Furthermore, they were disenchanted because nurses' training still focused heavily on "service to the patient" rather than on a comprehensive professional education. This was far removed from what the Nightingale Plan had proposed for aspiring nurses.

By 1940 thousands of self-taught "practical nurses" were working to meet the needs of the country. However, they lacked the education and experience that could be obtained only under supervision in an established program. They could not really be called practical/vocational nurses nor could they be licensed by the states. In fact, few states had even established minimal standards for the practice of practical/vocational nursing. Only nineteen states and one territory had passed or even considered legislation dealing with practical/vocational nursing. Licensure of the practical/vocational nurse was mandatory in only one state by the end of 1945. Many job descriptions and titles were used in referring to the work done by the practical/vocational nurse. There was no agreement on the duties, the role, or the responsibility of these people. These facts and the absence of standards and licensing practices created difficulties.

A quarter century after the end of World War I, the demand for trained nurses once again escalated due to the outbreak of the Second World War. The Cadet Nurse Corps was established to provide nursing education and training. The corps provided an abbreviated training program designed to meet the needs of the war effort. Additionally, federally subsidized programs in nursing were developed and implemented to offer women and, for the first time, men an education and career in nursing while serving their country in the war. After the war, many of the nurses trained by these programs remained in military service. Prestige, pay, and the opportunity for advancement were much greater in the military service than for civilian nurses. Civilian nurses received low pay and worked long shifts under atrocious conditions in the major hospitals, particularly in the urban areas. These conditions in no way could attract those who became nurses as a result of the war and who, ironically, enjoyed a certain lifestyle that war invariably provides. As a result, the shortage of nurses in the United States and other countries worsened.

World War II had an enormous effect on nursing. For the first time, large numbers of women worked outside the home. In the process, they also became more independent and assertive. These changes in women and in society resulted in an increased emphasis on education. The war itself had identified a need for more nurses and had resulted in a knowledge explosion in medicine and technology, which broadened the role of nurses. After World War II, efforts were directed at upgrading nursing education. Schools of nursing were based on educational objectives and were increasingly developed in university and college settings, leading to degrees in nursing for both men and women.

Nursing has broadened in all areas since the 1950s, including practice in a wide variety of health care settings, the development of a body of knowledge specific to nursing, the conduct and publication of nursing research, and the recognition of the role of nursing in promoting wellness. Increased emphasis on the importance of nursing knowledge as the base for nursing practice has led to the growth of nursing as a profession and as a discipline.

The Postwar Era

The effects of World War I, the Great Depression, and World War II all highlighted the shortage in qualified nurses. Pressure was exerted on the state boards of nursing, which had licensure responsibility, to mandate requirements for nurses. State-administered licensing examinations were no longer considered adequate for the country's needs. The parochial state examinations were in no way standardized and allowed a wide spectrum of competence to enter nursing. National norms of competence were needed and quickly established.

In 1944 the U.S. Department of Vocational Education commissioned an intensive study of practical/vocational nursing tasks. The outcome of this study differentiated the tasks performed by the registered nurse. As a result of this study, individual state boards of nursing began to specify the duties that could be accomplished by both groups of nurses.

The characteristics of health care changed rapidly as health care became an industry. Growth and diversity became the major emphasis as the industry of health care became increasingly lucrative. The need for nurses, particularly well-educated nurses, increased at a rate much greater than could be provided.

Another event that influenced change in attitude about practical/vocational nursing was the 1965 position paper of the American Nurses Association. This position clearly defined two levels of nursing practice; that of the registered nurse and that of the technical nurse. The term *practical nurse* was not included in this position paper. However, even with the exclusion of the practical/vocational nurse in the position paper, practical/vocational nurses have proved their worth and provide excellent bedside nursing skills in many areas of service.

The practical nurse provides valuable nursing interventions under the supervision of a registered nurse or physician.

The nursing organizations continued to deliberate on the future of nursing as a profession. In 1965 the American Nursing Association (ANA) took the position that nursing education should take place in institutions of learning within the general system of education, much as Robb and Nutting had proposed in 1903. Their position paper further delineated that the minimum preparation for a beginning professional nurse should be a baccalaureate degree in nursing and that the minimum education for technical nursing practice should be an associate degree in nursing. Assistants to nurses, they said, should have preservice programs in vocational education rather than just on-the-job training. This position has had a profound effect. Since 1965 many hospital-based nursing programs have been disbanded and an increasing number of baccalaureate and associate degree programs have been established in colleges and universities. The intent is obviously to change the trend from "training" nurses to "educating" nurses.

DEFINITIONS OF NURSING

The word *nurse* originated from the Latin word *nutrix*, meaning to nourish. Definitions of nurse and nursing describe one who nourishes, fosters, and protects; a person prepared to take care of the sick, injured, and aged people. However, the expanding roles and functions of the nurse in today's society have made any one definition too limited. It is no longer possible to say "a nurse is a nurse is a nurse." This section offers several definitions that provide a broad perspective of nursing.

In 1973, the International Council of Nurses adopted a definition of nursing written by Virginia Henderson. The basic belief of the definition is that the nurse is to provide assistance to a person in performing activities that contribute to health or aids in its recovery, that he would perform without assistance if he had the strength, will, and knowledge. In addition, the nurse is to do these activities in such a way, so the person may gain independence as quickly as possible.

The American Nurses Association (ANA) Committee on Education issued a position paper that broadly defined nursing as an independent profession. In summary, this position paper emphasizes that nursing is a helping profession that provides services that contribute to the health and well-being of people. The critical elements of professional nursing are care, cure, and coordination. Two important inclusions in this definition are professional nursing's responsibility for the health and welfare of communities, and the participation in programs of illness prevention and health maintenance.

These concepts and beliefs were expanded by ANA in 1980 in *Nursing: A Social Policy Statement,* which defined nursing practice as "the diagnosis and treatment of human responses to actual or potential health problems." This definition further legitimized the assessment and analysis of signs and symptoms and the use of nursing knowledge to implement and evaluate nursing actions taken to meet needs for potential or actual health problems.

In all of the definitions, the central focus is the person receiving care (who may be called either the patient or the client), and includes the physical, emotional, social, and spiritual dimensions of that person. Nursing is no longer considered to be primarily concerned with illness care; the concepts and definitions have expanded to include the prevention of illness, the promotion of wellness, and the maintenance of health for individuals, families, and communities.

A Profession and a Discipline

As definitions of nursing have expanded to describe more clearly the roles and actions of nurses, increased attention has focused on nursing as a profession and as a discipline. Nursing is gaining recognition as a profession based on the criteria that a profession must have:

- A well-defined body of knowledge
- A strong service orientation
- Recognized authority by a professional group
- A code of ethics
- A professional organization that sets standards
- Ongoing research
- Autonomy

A discipline has a specific and unique body of knowledge that uses existing and new knowledge to solve problems creatively and meet human needs within ever-changing boundaries. To be considered a discipline, certain criteria must be met:

- An impressive body of lasting works
- Suitable techniques
- Concerns that are relevant to human activities
- Relevant traditions that inspire future knowledge development
- Considerable scholarly recognition and achievement

Nursing involves specialized skills and application of knowledge based on education that has both theoretical and clinical components. Nurses uphold standards set forth by professional organizations and follow an established code of ethics. The concerns of nursing focus on human responses to actual or potential health problems and are increasingly focused on wellness, an area of caring that encompasses nursing's unique knowledge and abilities. Nursing is rich in tradition. Furthermore, it is increasingly being recognized as scholarly, with academic qualifications, research, and publications specific to nursing becoming more widely accepted and respected.

Nursing has evolved through history from a technical service to a person-centered process that affects the lives of others to allow maximizing of potential in all human dimensions. This has been an active process, as the profession and the discipline of nursing have developed by using lessons from the past to gain knowledge for practice in the present and in the future.

Aims of Nursing

The four broad aims of nursing practice can be identified from the definitions of nursing, which include wellness promotion, the prevention of illness, restoring of health, and facilitating coping.

To meet these aims, the nurse uses knowledge and skills to give care in a variety of traditional and expanding roles. The primary role of the nurse as caregiver is given shape and substance by the interrelated roles of communicator, teacher, counselor, leader, researcher, and advocate. These roles, as well as expanded career roles and functions of nurses, are defined in the tables listed in this section. Activities within the roles are carried out by the nurse in many different settings, including hospitals, nursing homes, clinics, offices, mobile units, and the home. Of these settings, care is increasingly provided out of the hospital and in the community. These activities are directed toward maximizing wellness for the patient and his or her family.

Promoting Wellness

Wellness is a state of human functioning that may be defined as the achievement of one's maximum attainable potential. The American Hospital Association in its description of wellness includes the essential aspect of enhancing the quality of life as a wellness objective. This enhancement is attained through activities that continually improve the person's physical, mental, emotional, and spiritual well-being.

Nurses promote wellness by maximizing strengths that are specific and individualized within each person. Wellness is an essential part of each of the other aims of nursing, with identification and analysis of patient strengths a component of preventing illness, restoring health, and facilitating coping with disability or death. Every patient, no matter how ill, has strengths. The nurse identifies and uses these strengths to help the patient reach maximum function and quality of life or meet death with dignity.

Wellness promotion is the framework for nursing activities. The patient's self-awareness, health awareness, wellness skills, and use of resources are all considered as the nurse provides care.

Through knowledge and skill, the nurse:

- Facilitates decisions about lifestyle that enhance the quality of life and encourages acceptance of responsibility for one's own health
- Increases health awareness by assisting in the understanding that health is more than just not being ill, and by teaching that certain behaviors and factors can contribute to or diminish wellness
- Teaches wellness skills by promoting decision making so that self-care activities maximize achievement of goals that are realistic and attainable, and by serving as a role model
- Encourages the use of wellness resources by providing information and referrals

Preventing Illness

The objective of illness-prevention activities is to reduce the risk of illness, to promote good health habits, and to maintain the individual's optimal functioning. Nurses primarily promote health by teaching and by personal examples. Such activities include the following:

- Educational programs in areas such as prenatal care for pregnant women, smoking-cessation programs, and stress reduction seminars
- Community programs and resources that encourage healthy lifestyles, including aerobic exercise classes, swimnastics, and physical fitness programs
- Literature and television information on diet, exercise, and the importance of good health habits
- Health assessments in institutions, clinics, and community settings that identify areas of strength and the potential for illness

Restoring Health

Activities to restore health encompass those most traditionally considered to be the nurse's responsibility. This area focuses on the individual with an illness but ranges from early detection of a disease to rehabilitation and teaching during recovery. Activities include:

- Providing direct care of the person who is ill by such measures as providing physical care, administering medications, and carrying out procedures and treatments
- Performing diagnostic measurements and examinations that detect an illness
- Referring questions and abnormal findings to other health care providers as appropriate
- Planning, teaching, and carrying out rehabilitation for illnesses such as heart attacks, arthritis, and strokes
- Working in mental health and chemical-dependency programs

Facilitating Coping

Although the major focus of health care is promoting, maintaining, or restoring health, these goals cannot always be met. Nurses also facilitate patient and family coping with altered function, life crisis, and death. Altered function results in a decrease in an individual's ability to carry out activities of daily living and expected roles. Nurses can facilitate an optimal level of function through maximizing strengths and potentials, teaching, and knowledge of and referral to community support systems. Nurses provide care to both patients and families during a terminal illness, and they do so in hospitals, long-term nursing facilities, and homes. Nurses are also becoming more active in hospice programs, which assist individuals and their families in preparing for death and in living as comfortably as possible until death occurs. Table 1–2 discusses the various roles and functions of nurses.

NURSING EDUCATION

 ASK YOURSELF

With the various levels of nursing practice and the different levels and amount of education required for each, how does the nursing profession explain this to the health care consumer? How would you explain the differences when questioned by a patient or family member? What about the differences in the scope of practice? How will future nursing trends affect the various levels of education and practice?

TABLE 1–2

Roles and Functions of Nurses

Role	Function
Caregiver	The provision of care to patients that combines both the art and the science of nursing in meeting physical, emotional, intellectual, sociocultural, and spiritual needs. As a caregiver, the nurse integrates the roles of communicator, teacher, counselor, and leader; researcher; advocate to promote well-ness through activities that prevent illness, restore health, and facilitate coping with disability or death. The role of caregiver is the primary role of the nurse.
Communicator	The use of effective interpersonal and therapeutic communica-tion skills to establish and maintain helping relationships with patients of all ages in a wide variety of health care settings.
Teacher	The use of communication skills to assess, implement, and evaluate individualized teaching plans to meet learning needs of patients and their families.
Counselor	The use of therapeutic interpersonal communication skills to provide information, make appropriate referrals, and facilitate the patient's problem-solving and decision-making skills.
Leader	The assertive, self-confident practice of nursing when provid-ing care, effecting change, and functioning with groups.
Researcher	The participation in or conduct of research to increase knowledge in nursing and improve patient care.
Advocate	The protection of human or legal rights and securing of care for all patients based on the belief that patients have the right to make informed decisions about their own health and lives.

Levels of Education

Educational preparation for nursing practice currently involves several different types of programs. Students may choose to enter a practical/ vocational nursing program and be licensed as a licensed practical nurse (LPN) or licensed vocational nurse (LVN), or they may enter a diploma, an associate degree, or a baccalaureate program to be licensed as a registered nurse (RN). State laws in the United States and in some provinces of Canada recognize both the LPN or LVN and RN as having the proper credentials to practice nursing, although the responsibilities are different for the two levels. Graduate programs are also available in nursing, providing master's and doctoral degrees.

A major issue in nursing involves educational preparation. The multiple educational preparations are confusing to institutions employing nurses, to consumers of health care services, and to nurses themselves. Nursing organizations are working hard to answer questions such as: "What is technical nursing?" and "What is professional nursing?" as well as, "Should graduates of all programs take the same kind of licensing examination and have the same title?" It is imperative that these questions be resolved promptly through the collaborative efforts of nursing education and practice.

The following section discusses education for LPNs and RNs, as well as graduate nursing education, continuing education for nurses, and in-service education.

Practical and Vocational Nursing Education

Practical nursing was established to teach graduates to give bedside nursing care to patients. Schools for practical nursing programs are located in such varied settings as high schools, technical or vocational schools, community colleges, or independent agencies. Many programs are one-year programs divided into one-third classroom and two-thirds clinical laboratory hours. On completion of the program, graduates are eligible to take the National Council Licensure Examination (NCLEX-PN) for licensure as a licensed practical nurse (LPN) or licensed vocational nurse (LVN). In Canada, some provinces offer a similar program for practitioners called registered nursing assistants.

LPNs work under the direction of a physician or RN to give direct patient care, assist in patient education, manage team nursing patient care delivery, supervise unlicensed assistive personnel (UAP), focus on meeting health care needs in hospitals, nursing homes, urgent care centers, freestanding health care agencies, clinics, transitional care units, skilled nursing facilities, hospice care, and home health agencies.

Development of Practical/Vocational Nursing. The first school for practical nurse training started in Brooklyn, New York, in 1892 and was conducted under the auspices of the Young Women's Christian

Association (YWCA). The Ballard School, as it was known, was approximately three months in duration and trained its students to care for the chronically ill, the invalid, children, and the elderly. The main emphasis was on home care and included cooking, nutrition, basic science, and basic nursing procedures. Graduates of this program were referred to as attendant nurses.

Two other programs were started, and they were patterned after the Ballard School. In 1907 the Thompson Practical Nursing School opened in Brattleboro, Vermont, and in 1918 the Household Nursing Association School of Attendant Nursing (later changed to the Shepard-Gill School of Practical Nursing) opened in Boston. The focus of these programs continued to be on home nursing care and light housekeeping duties. Hospital experience was not a part of the training in the early programs. The Thompson School is still in operation and continues to be accredited by the National League for Nursing (NLN). Practical nursing programs developed slowly during the first half of the twentieth century. A total of thirty-six schools opened during this period.

There were few controls, little educational planning, and minimal supervision of practical nursing schools before 1940. The increased demand for nursing services brought on by World War II and the postwar years and the excellent bedside nursing care evidenced by the practical nurse resulted in the opening of 260 practical/vocational nursing programs between 1948 and 1954. These programs varied in administrative design. Some were affiliated with hospitals or chronic care institutions, whereas others aligned themselves with private agencies or private schools. Their commitment was meeting the needs of the sick. Students in these programs provided nursing services while they were obtaining their education and training. This apprentice training emphasized vocational/technical education. The allocation of federal funds for training practical/vocational nurses helped recruit men and women.

Practical nursing programs were increasing rapidly. The need to establish standards again became a major issue. The Association of Practical Nurse Schools was founded in 1941 and was dedicated exclusively to practical nursing. Its membership was multidisciplinary and included licensed practical nurses, registered nurses, physicians, hospital and nursing home administrators, students, and public figures. Together they planned the first standard curriculum for practical nursing. By 1942 they saw the need to change the name to the National Association of Practical Nurse Education (NAPNE). They broadened their focus to include education and practice and established an accrediting service for schools of practical/vocational nursing in 1945. The association changed its name in 1959 to the National Association for Practical Nurse Education and Service (NAPNES).

In 1949 the National Federation of Licensed Practical Nurses (NFLPN) was founded by Lillian Kuster. This association is the official membership organization for licensed practical and vocational nurses, and membership is limited to LVNs and LPNs.

These two organizations, the NAPNES and the NFLPN, set standards for practical/vocational nursing practice, promote and protect the interests of practical/vocational nurses, and educate and inform the general public about practical/vocational nursing.

In 1961 the NLN broadened its scope of service because of the growth of practical/vocational nursing programs. The NLN established a Department of Practical Nursing Programs and developed an accreditation service for these programs, which is now called the Council of Practical Nursing Programs.

For twenty years both the NLN and NAPNES provided accreditation services. Nursing programs had the option of selecting either organization from which to seek accreditation. In recent years, however, the NAPNES has discontinued this service.

Accreditation of a program differs from program approval. An **approved program** is one that meets minimum standards set by the respective state agency responsible for overseeing educational programs. The state seeks to ensure that a given program, for example, meets the needs of the student, has adequate course content and qualified faculty, is of sufficient length, has adequate facilities, and provides clinical experience. All these elements are needed for licensure. The state also ensures that the welfare of the public is protected by maintaining minimum standards. Approval is required for the program to operate. **Accreditation** involves the administration of a program voluntarily seeking a review by a given organization to determine whether the program meets the preestablished criteria of that organization. Many times the standards established by professional accrediting organizations are far higher than those established by the state. Although graduates of nonaccredited programs can take the licensure examination required in most states, accreditation is extremely important when programs seek federal funding.

Practical/vocational nursing programs continued to proliferate, and by the 1990–1991 school year, 1,125 practical/vocational nursing programs in the United States produced 38,100 graduates. Nursing programs are still offered by various organizations, such as high schools, trade or technical schools, hospitals, community colleges, colleges and universities, and private education agencies. Health care corporations such as the Gallen Health Institutes, Inc. also offer practical/vocational nursing programs. However, they must all meet minimum state standards. The length of the programs is usually 12 to 18 months, with a focus on nursing skills and theory that are correlated with clinical practice. On completing the program, the graduate is eligible to take the National Council Licensing Examination for Practical Nursing (NCLEX-PN).

Creative educational programs in nursing today offer various approaches to educating student practical/vocational nurses. The combination of practical/vocational nurse education with associate degree programs in two-year colleges is available. At the successful completion of the first academic year, the student can either exit and take the licensure examination for practical/vocational nursing or continue for another year and earn an associate degree in nursing, becoming eligible to take the licensure examination for registered nursing. Many other programs offering other combinations of education and degrees are available throughout the United States. Many states have some type of articulation plan.

Licensing the Practical/Vocational Nurse. Licensing laws have been passed throughout the states to protect the public from unqualified persons practicing in almost any field or profession. Every state and the District of Columbia, American Samoa, the Northern Mariana Islands, and the Virgin Islands have licensing laws that apply to the practical/vocational nurse. These laws are put into effect through various state agencies, usually the state boards of nursing and the Nurse Practice Acts of the respective states.

Licensing for practical nurses in the United States began in 1914 when the state legislature in Mississippi passed the first laws pertaining to that group. This followed the passage of laws on licensing registered nurses by eleven years. The passage of such laws governing practical/vocational nursing in other states was slow in coming. Only six states passed such laws between 1920 and 1940. This may have been because there were not many practical nurses' training programs initiated during that period. After the outbreak of World War II and the opening of a large number of practical/vocational nurses' training programs, all the states were forced to pass legislation concerning the licensing of practical/vocational nurses. By 1955 all states had passed laws in this area in consonance with the standards set by NAPNE. The State Board Test Pool of the NLN Education Committee established a testing mechanism for all states and administered the examination several times a year throughout the United States. Graduates of a state-approved practical/vocational nursing education program were eligible to take the examination and, if they passed, became licensed practical nurses (LPNs) or licensed vocational nurses (LVNs), as they are called in Texas and California. Each state established its own required passing score on the examination.

Currently, graduates of a state-approved LPN/LVN education program are eligible to take the NCLEX-PN. On completing the examination with a "pass" score, the graduate is issued a license to practice as an LPN or an LVN.

Licensing laws for nursing are now established in all states. It is the individual's responsibility to be informed regarding licensure in the state in which he or she resides, or intends, to practice. Interstate endorsement (reciprocity between states) exists, and licensing for practice in other states can be obtained without repeating the NCLEX-PN if resident state requirements are met.

Roles and Responsibilities. The stated objectives for practical/vocational nursing practice are: to acquire the specialized knowledge and skills needed to meet the health needs of patients in a variety of settings; to be a graduate of a state-approved practical/vocational nursing program; to take and pass the NCLEX-PN examination; and to acquire a state license to practice.

To accomplish these objectives, students must assume responsibility for their own education, intensive study, and dedication to duty. Organizing one's time effectively helps accomplish these objectives and ultimately assures the patient of safe and competent care.

Practical/vocational nursing is the activity of providing specific services to patients under the direct supervision of a licensed physician or dentist and/or RN. The services are provided in a structured setting surrounding the caring for the sick, the rehabilitation of the sick and injured, and the prevention of sickness and injury (Table 1–3). This definition is adapted from the NAPNES and several states' Nurse Practice Acts.

The unique function of the nurse is to assist individuals, sick or well, in the performance of those activities contributing to health, to their recovery, or to a peaceful death—activities that patients would perform unaided if they had the necessary strength, will, or knowledge—and if

TABLE 1–3

Characteristics, Roles, and Responsibilities of the Practical/Vocational Nurse

- Being a responsible and accountable member of the health care team
- Maintaining a current license
- Practicing within the scope of the Nurse Practice Act
- Practicing under the supervision of a medical physician, RN, osteopathic physician, or dentist
- Participating in continuing education activities
- Being an effective member of the health care team
- Using the nursing process to meet patients' needs
- Promoting and maintaining health, preventing disease, and encouraging and assisting in rehabilitation
- Maintaining a professional appearance
- Subscribing to recognized ethical practices
- Performing within legal parameters
- Participating in activities of professional organizations
- Assisting in developing the role of the licensed practical/vocational nurse for tomorrow

feasible to do this in such a way as to help patients gain independence as rapidly as possible. The practical/vocational nurse is educated to be a responsible member of a health care team, performing basic therapeutic, rehabilitative, and preventive care for anyone who needs it.

In 1981 NAPNES issued the following statement of responsibilities required for practice as a practical/vocational nurse:

- Recognizes the LPN/LVN's role in the health care delivery system and articulates that role with those of other health care team members
- Maintains accountability for one's own nursing practice within the ethical and legal framework
- Serves as a patient advocate
- Accepts their role in maintaining, developing standards of practice in providing health care
- Seeks further growth through educational opportunities

The role of the practical/vocational nurse is not new within the health care delivery system. The role and responsibilities have expanded from bathing patients and light housekeeping to performing skilled tasks needed to provide health care to people within the wellness/ illness continuum.

The role of the LPN/LVN continues to evolve. This evolution is influenced by various states' Nurse Practice Acts, individual changes within the health care agencies, the availability of health care workers, and the needs of the patients. The practical/vocational nurse is finding a career in hospitals, clinics, outpatient agencies, home health agencies, long-term care facilities, insurance companies, physician offices, and the military service. The blend of nursing history and today's health care delivery system sets the foundation for the career of an LPN/LVN.

Registered Nursing Education

Three primary types of educational programs lead to licensure as an RN. In the United States, these types are (1) diploma, (2) associate degree, and (3) baccalaureate programs. Graduates of all types of programs take the same RN licensing examination. In the United States, graduates take the NCLEX-RN examination, and graduates of Canadian schools take the Canadian Nurses Association Testing Service examination. Although both are national examinations, they are administered by, and the nurse is licensed in, each state or province. It is illegal to practice nursing unless one has a license verifying completion of an accredited (by the state or province) program in nursing and has passed the licensing examination. Nurses gain legal rights to practice nursing in another state or province by applying to that state's or province's board of nursing and receiving reciprocal licensure.

Diploma in Nursing. Many nurses practicing in the United States received their basic nursing education in three-year, hospital-based diploma schools of nursing. The first schools of nursing established to educate nurses were diploma programs, and until the 1960s, they were the major source of graduates. In recent years the number of diploma programs has greatly decreased.

Current graduates of diploma programs have a sound foundation of the biologic and social sciences, with a strong emphasis on clinical experience in direct patient care. Graduates work in acute, long-term, and ambulatory health care facilities.

Associate Degree in Nursing. Associate degree nursing education is based on a research project carried out in the 1950s. At that time, a shortage of nurses existed, and the project was created to meet the needs of society by preparing nurses in less time than was required in diploma programs. The emphasis of this type of program was education instead of service.

Currently, most associate degree programs are offered in community junior colleges. These two-year educational programs attract more men, more minorities, and more nontraditional students than do the other types of programs. Associate degree education prepares nurses to give care to patients in structured settings, including hospitals, long-term care, and home health. Graduates of these programs are technically skilled and well prepared to carry out nursing roles and functions. Competencies of the associate degree nurse for entry into practice, as defined by the National League for Nursing (NLN), are listed in this chapter.

Baccalaureate in Nursing. The first baccalaureate nursing programs were established in the United States and Canada in the early 1900s. However, the number of programs and the number of enrolling students did not increase markedly until the 1960s. (Most graduates receive a bachelor of science in nursing (BSN) degree and, hence, are referred to having a BSN throughout this section.)

The increase in number of programs and student enrollment is the result of recommendations made by ANA, NLN, and CNA that the entry level for professional practice be at the baccalaureate level. Although nurses with a BSN practice in a wide variety of settings, the four-year degree is required for many administrative, managerial, and community health positions.

In BSN programs, the major in nursing is built on a general education base with concentration on nursing at the upper level. Students acquire knowledge of theory and practice related to nursing and other disciplines, provide nursing care to individuals and groups, work with members of the health care team, use research to improve practice, and have a foundation for graduate study. Nurses who graduate from a diploma or associate degree program and wish to complete requirements for a BSN may choose to enroll in an RN to BSN program or may complete requirements through an external degree program. Characteristics of the graduate of the baccalaureate program in nursing as defined by NLN are listed in this chapter.

Graduate Education in Nursing. The two levels of graduate education in nursing are the master's and doctoral degrees. A master's degree in nursing prepares the graduate to function in educational settings, in managerial roles, as clinical specialists, and as nurse practitioners. Nurses with doctoral degrees meet requirements for academic advancement and are prepared to carry out research necessary to advance nursing theory and practice.

Continuing Education

Continuing education is defined as those professional development experiences designed to enrich the nurse's contribution to health. Formal continuing education through courses, seminars, and workshops is offered by colleges, hospitals, voluntary agencies, and private groups. In some states, continuing education is required to maintain licensure.

Many hospitals and health care agencies provide education and training for employees of their institution or organization. This is called in-service education and is designed to increase the knowledge and skills of the nursing staff. Programs might involve learning a nursing skill or how to use new equipment.

NURSING ORGANIZATIONS

One of the criteria of a profession is having a professional organization that sets standards for practice and education. Nursing meets this criterion. Professional organizations also are concerned with current issues in nursing and health care, and influence health care legislation. The benefits of belonging to a professional nursing organization include networking with colleagues, having a voice in the legislation affecting nursing, and keeping current with trends and issues in nursing.

National Organizations

North America has several major professional organizations for nurses: ANA, CNA, NAPNES, NFLPN, and NLN. The ANA is the professional organization for RNs in the United States. Founded in the late 1800s, its members are state nurses associations, with individual nurses belonging to the state organization. ANA establishes standards of practice, encourages research to advance nursing practice, represents nursing through legislative actions, and supports the National Student Nurses' Association (NSNA).

CNA is the national nursing association for RNs in Canada. CNA has provincial organizations supported by local districts. CNA supports the same goals as ANA—to improve standards of health, to foster high standards of nursing, and to promote the professional development and welfare of nurses. CNA has also been active in nursing education, licensing, and registration for nurses.

NAPNES, the National Association for Practical Nurse Education and Service, Inc., was organized in 1941 and is the oldest organization dedicated exclusively to practical/vocational nursing. The purpose of NAPNES is to promote an understanding of practical/vocational nursing through establishing and maintaining educational standards for practical/vocational nursing preparation. It provides opportunities for LPNs/LVNs to participate in continuing education programs. NAPNES publishes standards of nursing practice, and its official publication, the *Journal of Practical Nursing,* provides its members with information on organizational activities. Membership is open to licensed practical/ vocational nurses, practical/vocational nursing students, faculty and school directors, health care agency personnel, physicians, and lay-persons interested in promoting practical/vocational nursing.

The purpose of NFLPN is to promote the practice of practical/ vocational nursing and it is dedicated to maintaining high standards of nursing education for practical/vocational nursing. It was founded in 1949, and its membership is limited to practical/vocational nurses. NFLPN was influential in changing the membership composition of state boards of nursing examiners to include a practical/vocational nurse. The activities of the association include defining ethical conduct, providing standards and scope of practice for practical/vocational nursing, and sponsoring educational programs that provide continuing education credit.

NLN is an organization open to all people interested in nursing, including nurses, non-nurses, and agencies. Established in 1952, its objective is to foster the development and improvement of all nursing services and nursing education. The following are the major activities of NLN:

- Conducts one of the largest professional testing services in the United States, including pre-entrance testing for potential students and achievement testing to measure student progress
- Sponsors continuing education workshops and seminars nationwide
- Serves as the primary source of research data about nursing education; conducts annual surveys of schools and new RNs
- Provides voluntary accreditation for educational programs in nursing

The national organizations for student nurses are NSNA in the United States and the Canadian University Nursing Student Organization in Canada. Members are students enrolled in nursing education programs. Programs and activities focus on professional development and health care.

International Organizations

The ICN, founded in 1899, was the first international organization of professional women, with nurses from both the United States and

Canada among the charter members. By sharing a commitment to maintaining high standards of nursing service and nursing education and by promoting ethics, ICN provides a way for national nursing organizations to work together. The ICN (1973) Code for Nurses stated, "The need for nursing is universal. Inherent in nursing is respect for life, dignity and rights of man. It is unrestricted by considerations of nationality, race, creed, color, age, sex, politics, or social status."

Specialty Organizations

A wide variety of nursing organizations currently is available to nurses. These organizations provide information on specific areas of nursing, often have publications directed toward the specialty area of nursing, and may be involved in certification activities. The following examples illustrate the variety of organizations:

American Association of Critical Care Nurses
Association of Operating Room Nurses
American Indian Nurses' Association
Canadian Gerontological Nursing Association
National Black Nurses' Association, Inc.
Nurses' Christian Fellowship
American Public Health Association

Participation in professional organizations and associations can be an important factor in your development as a nurse. Active involvement can provide opportunities for professional and personal growth through the variety of services offered. An added benefit is the opportunity to meet nursing leaders and share ideas about health care issues and nursing trends, and to actively network with nursing colleagues.

NURSE PRACTICE AND LICENSING

Nurse practice acts are laws established in each state (United States) and province (Canada) to regulate the practice of nursing. They are broadly worded and vary among jurisdictions, but all of them have certain elements in common. In general, they:

- Are designed to protect the public by defining the legal scope of nursing practice, excluding untrained or unlicensed people from practicing nursing
- Create a state board of nursing or regulatory body having the authority to make and enforce rules and regulations concerning the nursing profession

- Define important terms and activities in nursing, including legal requirements and titles for RNs and LPNs/LVNs
- Establish criteria for the education and licensure of nurses

The board of nursing for each state or province is given legal authority to approve taking the licensing examination to graduates of approved schools of nursing. The individual who successfully meets the requirements for licensure is then given a license to practice nursing in the state or province. The license, which must be renewed annually, is valid during the life of the holder and is registered in the state or province. The license and the right to practice nursing can be denied, revoked, or suspended for professional misconduct (e.g., incompetence, negligence, chemical impairment, or criminal actions).

As nursing roles continue to expand, and as issues in nursing are resolved, nurse practice acts will reflect those changes. It is essential that nurses are knowledgeable of the specific nurse practice act under which they practice.

Nursing in Transition

Nursing changes constantly in response to the needs and resources of society as a whole. Nursing also changes in response to factors such as definitions of nursing, aims of nursing, educational levels of nursing, and expanded practice roles. Current issues and trends in nursing briefly discussed in this section are new directions in nursing, changes in patient needs, expanded technology, and increasing autonomy. These are complex subjects and the information provided is only intended to serve as an introduction (Table 1–4).

TABLE 1–4

Expanded Career Roles and Functions of Nurses

Title	Description
Clinical nurse specialist (e.g., enterostomal therapist, geriatrics, infection control, medical-surgical, maternal-child, oncology, quality assurance, nursing process)	A nurse with an advanced degree, education, or experience who is considered to be an expert in a specialized area of nursing; carries out direct patient care, consultation, teaching patients, families and staff; and conducting research

Table 1-4 *continued*

Nurse practitioner	A nurse with an advanced degree, certified for a special area or age of patient care; works in a variety of health care settings or in independent practice to make health assessments and deliver primary care
Nurse anesthetist	A nurse who completes a course of study in anesthesia school; carries out preoperative visits and assessments, administers and monitors anesthesia during surgery, and evaluates postoperative status of patients
Nurse midwife	A nurse who completes a program in midwifery; provides prenatal and postnatal care and delivers babies to women with uncomplicated pregnancies
Nurse educator	A nurse, usually with an advanced degree, who teaches in educational or clinical settings; teaches theoretical knowledge and clinical skills; conducts research
Nurse administrator	A nurse who functions at various levels of management in health care settings; responsible for the management and administration of resources and personnel involved in giving patient care
Nurse researcher	A nurse with an advanced degree who conducts research relevant to the definition and improvement of nursing practice and education
Nurse entrepreneur	A nurse, usually with an advanced degree, who may manage a clinic or health-related business, conduct research, provide education, or serve as an advisor or consultant to institutions, political agencies, or businesses

New Directions in Nursing

Currently, there is a shortage of nurses prepared at advanced levels (i.e., master's and doctoral degrees) and those with the knowledge and skills to meet the complex needs of the patient in the home setting. Various factors have been identified as responsible for this shortage, including a change in the health care needs of patients, economic conditions affecting the setting in which care is given, and career mobility.

Individuals requiring care are more acutely ill but spend less time within the hospital setting as a result of health care reimbursement plans. This has resulted in a demand for nursing care in community settings. With advanced education and expanded roles, nurses are taking advantage of career mobility to move into management, educational, and community settings. In addition, nurse practitioners are increasingly establishing independent practices where they diagnose and treat illnesses. Nurses also have increased autonomy (i.e., freedom to regulate their work behavior) in making decisions about the care of others and are being paid better for their knowledge and skill.

Changes in Patient Needs. Changes such as the trend toward shorter hospital care have created new patient needs, and thus new opportunities for nursing. Patient education is an important aspect of care—teaching patients and their families how to care for the patients after dismissal from the hospital often begins before or on admission. Consideration of the health care needs of the patient and the family in the home setting is a major component of planning patient care. It is essential to maintain continuity in care between the nurse in the hospital and the nurse in the home setting. In addition, patients who require hospital care are increasingly older and/or acutely ill. The complex needs of the patient during the acute stage of illness or injury while in the hospital setting requires nursing knowledge and skill to provide not only "high-tech" but also "high-touch" care.

Another aspect of changes in patient needs is the increasing population of older people who require both wellness promotion and health restoration. Other changes in patient needs that require nursing consideration involve the homeless, indigent, and people with acquired immunodeficiency syndrome. These groups, as well as others, require innovative nursing care to meet special needs.

Expanded Technology. Both technologic advances and increased autonomy affect nursing practice today. It is impossible to visit a health care setting of any type without being aware of the rapid advances that have been made in technology. Diagnostic procedures, inpatient and outpatient surgical procedures, intensive care units, and patient care units are all heavily based on high-tech concepts and machines. These machines go home with the patient, where ventilators, kidney dialysis machines, intravenous fluids, and a wide variety of monitors are becoming more common. The nurse must continually update knowledge and skills to use technology to give safe, individualized care. In addition, computerization in a wide variety of applications has become commonplace in health care, providing more accurate assessments, monitoring infusion rates, and providing documentation and care plan capabilities (Table 1–5).

Increasing Autonomy. Nursing interventions—the activities nurses carry out as caregivers—are also in transition. Nursing autonomy has increased and the special role of the nurse in providing care has been recognized. It is important to realize that with authority to carry out actions also comes responsibility for one's actions. Even if an action is carried out on the direct order of a physician, the nurse is still responsible for using critical thinking based on knowledge to provide safe care.

Traditionally, nursing actions have been divided into three categories:

Dependent Nursing Actions. Those activities that the nurse does based on physician orders are considered dependent nursing actions. Even dependent actions (e.g., administering prescribed medications) require knowledge and skill as well as the legal responsibility to question any order that is inappropriate.

Interdependent Nursing Actions. Interdependent or collaborative nursing actions are those activities that the nurse carries out in collaboration with other members of the health care team. Examples include monitoring the patient for side effects of medications or for changes in the results of diagnostic tests, and reporting findings that indicate increased risk for illness to the appropriate person.

Independent Nursing Actions. Activities that the nurse orders and carries out based on assessment, knowledge, and judgment are independent nursing actions. A wide range of activities is included in this area, including health assessments, nursing diagnoses and care plans, teaching, and counseling.

The distinctions among these categories are blurring as nurses increase educational levels and legal authority to diagnose and treat

TABLE 1–5

Computer Applications in Nursing

The National Council Licensure Examination for Nurses

Since April 1994, The National Council of State Boards of Nursing Examination, known as the National Council Licensure Examination (NCLEX), has been administered via computer. Previously, graduate nurses in all states took a paper-and-pencil examination that was offered only twice a year within a two-day period. Now graduates may take the examination year-round at their convenience in a one-day time frame. The NCLEX is administered at more than 200 locations nationwide, which is a fourfold increase over the previous examination sites.

The test is written using the computerized adaptive testing (CAT) method, which uses computer technology and measurement theory. Standard multiple-choice questions are used, but each candidate's test is different. Questions are answered and the computer calculates a competence index based on all this and earlier answers. Subsequent questions are selected by the computer based on previous answers. The examination continues until a pass or fail decision is made. The graduate has up to five hours (including rest breaks) to complete the examination.

Candidates may not skip questions or return to previous questions because of the adaptive branching testing. Once an answer is given, the next questions are based on that answer. NCLEX candidates need not be skilled in computer use before taking the examination. A keyboard tutorial and practice exercise are given before the examination. The space bar and the enter key are the only two keys needed to take the examination.

The results of the examination are transmitted electronically on a daily basis to the National State Board Educational Testing Service. Pass/fail reports will be sent to the State Boards of Nursing for distribution to the candidate. Results may be known within one month; previously, testing results were not known until three months later.

The examination tests the knowledge, skills, and abilities needed to demonstrate the safe and effective practice of entry-level nursing. The test questions are written by nursing professionals and reviewed by a national panel of nursing experts.

illnesses. A major trend is toward nurse practitioners establishing practices in which they, in collaboration with a physician, independently provide care for patients of all ages. Whereas hospital-based nursing care is often primarily dependent on physician orders, home-based care is more independent and collaborative in meeting patient health care needs. Regardless of the type of intervention, independent nursing judgment is required as the intervention is carried out.

As nurses continue to define their own practice, the special and distinctive role of nursing in caring for others will become increasingly recognized.

TRADITIONS AND CEREMONIES IN NURSING

Historically, nursing has developed a number of rich traditions. Some of the traditions and ceremonies are being eliminated and others are being reviewed for their purpose and practicality. For example, the wearing of caps has been eliminated in most nursing education programs, and very few graduate nurses wear their caps. However, it is important to discuss the development of some of these traditions and their relationship to nursing practice.

The Nursing Uniform

The nursing uniform came from the special dress associated with the military and religious orders. The uniform has been significant to nursing partly because dress provides a strong nonverbal message about one's image. In the 1950s and 1960s, the nurse wearing the white uniform communicated confidence, professionalism, competence, and authority. Within the last two decades, nurses have employed a casual, and sometimes colorful uniform attire. Initially, the bright colors and various designs were limited to pediatric nurses however, now this type of uniform is worn by many nurses in various types of clinical practice settings. Some nurses working in critical care specialty areas such as ICU, CCU, ER, PACU, wear scrub attire and this type of uniform has proved to be more practical in these areas. Some of the identity of the starched, white uniform has been lost and nursing education and practice, hospital committees, and nurses have discussed various options and dress codes.

The uniforms of the early nursing years were long, starched, long sleeved, with detachable collars and cuffs. The complete uniform included a cape, usually navy blue with a red lining, that was worn as

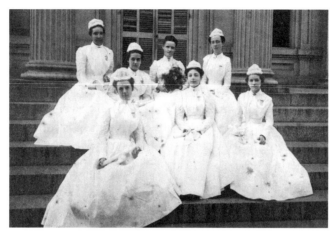

FIGURE 1–4 Graduating class (1900) of Touro Infirmary Training School for Nurses. *(Photo courtesy of Touro Infirmary Archives, New Orleans, LA)*

an outer garment during the winter. The New York Training School for Nurses at Bellevue Hospital was the first school to adopt a standard uniform for student nurses in 1876. This first student nurse uniform included a gingham apron worn in the morning hours and a white apron worn during the afternoon over a dark wool dress.

By the end of the nineteenth century, a regulation uniform had been adopted by most nursing education programs. Usually, the uniform consisted of a dress of white material, long sleeves with white cuffs, a white collar, and a cap. Corsets were worn beneath the uniforms and the student nurses' ankles were hidden from public view (Figure 1–4).

By the 1900s, the uniform became more functional and hemlines were raised. Pantsuits became acceptable during the 1960s and during this time some nurses were challenging wearing white uniforms in certain patient care areas. Pediatric and psychiatric nurses questioned the therapeutic effect of wearing white uniforms in these patient care areas. By the 1970s, in the psychiatric setting, it became acceptable for nurses to wear street clothes in patient care areas. The belief behind this move was that the nurses would be more approachable and would appear less threatening to psychiatric patients. Currently, uniform magazines and catalogs feature uniforms with a variety of styles. Athletic shoes are acceptable as standard uniform shoe wear in many facilities, and many nurses prefer clogs or clog-like shoes versus shoes that are enclosed. Many nurses prefer the comfort of scrubs in varying colors or a lab coat over street wear as their uniform of choice. The changes in attire have made it difficult for some consumers to identify the nurse because they are no longer identifiable by the uniform. The identification badge provides information but frequently does not include the person's full name.

Currently, there remains a controversy over appropriate nurses' attire, and it is recommended that nurses dress in attire that clearly distinguishes them as professional nurses. This issue of appropriate professional dress will remain controversial and requires collaboration and compromise.

The Nursing Cap

The nursing cap history is not documented very well. How the cap originated is unclear, but some historians believe it is connected to the influence of the religious orders. The Sisters of Charity of Saint Vincent de Paul, who established the first modern school of nursing in Paris in 1864, wore habits and some nursing historians believe that the cap was included as a part of the religious habit. Others believe that the cap originated at Kaiserwerth in Germany, where Florence Nightingale studied. There is strong discussion about the cap of the deaconesses of the Christian era, and the nun's veil; many say these were the beginning influences for the nurses' cap of the twentieth century. The veil was modified to become a cap and was associated with service to others. During the time of Florence Nightingale and Queen Victoria, it was appropriate for young ladies to have their heads covered during the day, consequently, the cap was viewed as appropriate attire for a young woman of the day. When Florence Nightingale was a student at Kaiserwerth, the cap was designed to cover the long hair that was very fashionable during the nineteenth century. Short hair was not acceptable for women during this time and the head covering was used to control the hair. The hair covering continued as a part of the cap in England and Europe. Hospital-based nursing education programs created their own cap as a symbol of that particular nursing program. The styles of the cap ranged from tall and wide, with a stiff, starched appearance, to small, lacy, ruffled pillboxes. Hairstyles changed and the size of the caps changed to meet the demands and preferences of the nurses.

The health care environment has changed and today the cap is not practical in many patient care areas. By the early 1980s, many hospitals were no longer requiring the cap as a part of the nurse's uniform. Many nursing education programs supported the hospitals, and did not require the cap as a part of the student uniform.

Some nursing education programs still have a capping ceremony, where the student receives a cap, but it is not required as a part of the student uniform.

Many nursing leaders support removing the cap as a required part of the nurse's uniform and a variety of reasons are provided: (1) the cap is no longer practical, given the expanded nursing roles of today; (2) wearing a cap discourages men from entering professional nursing; (3) the cap has a "handmaiden" image attached to it; (4) many nursing education programs no longer have a cap identified with their school; (5) the cap is difficult to keep clean and fresh.

The Nursing Pin

The nursing pin may have originated during the time of the Crusades. The Knights Hospitallers were among the Crusaders and their uniforms included a white cross, which was recognized in the Holy Land on the battlefields. The Maltese cross is an eight-pointed cross formed by four arrowheads. The eight points signified the beatitudes that the knights were expected to reflect in their charity works. The Maltese cross became a symbol of many groups who cared for the sick, including the United States Cadet Nurse Corps.

The symbolism of the pin is related to the traditions of the sixteenth century, when noblemen wore a coat of arms. This coat of arms was worn only by those who served their kings well and so it was associated with loyalty and courage. The distinction of wearing a coat of arms was extended to schools and it symbolized strength, wisdom, courage, and faith. Florence Nightingale adopted the Maltese cross as a symbol for the badge worn by the graduates of her nursing school.

Throughout the years, each nursing school adopted a pin unique to their school and it was awarded at graduation. Many of the first nursing schools in the United States were hospital based supported by religious associations and the cross was integrated in the design of the school pin. The first nursing school pin in the United States was created at Bellevue Hospital, and it was presented to the graduating class of 1880. Many nursing schools today still award the school pin during the graduation ceremonies, whereas others no longer offer the school pin.

Ceremonies

Historically, the premier ceremonies of nursing education have been the "pinning" and the "capping" ceremonies. Capping is not as popular today because most nursing education programs do not have caps and most nurses do not wear caps. The cap was given to students after they reached a particular point in the nursing program and, depending on the school, stripes were given later at various clinical or academic levels. The ceremony was especially planned and usually it was held in the church, with family and guests in attendance. After the caps were awarded, students were expected to wear them as a required part of the student nurse uniform.

The pinning ceremony in some schools was included with the graduation ceremony because it signified the completion of the nursing program, and the pin could only be worn by graduates.

The ceremony participants included the program director and the nursing faculty, and the graduates recited a nursing pledge, most frequently, the Nightingale pledge. The pinning ceremony was very significant and many nursing schools have continued this tradition today.

Although nursing educational preparation has moved into the collegiate environment, many of the traditional ceremonies have been discontinued. Many believe that the college commencement is the most appropriate ceremony to recognize nursing graduates at the completion of their respective educational programs. Hence, special recognition of students for particular areas of study are not included. In many of the larger university settings, various disciplines have separate ceremonies or an additional ceremony for their members.

KEY POINTS

- Nursing has always involved caring; the role of the nurse as caregiver has been present since early civilization.
- Definitions of nursing have changed and expanded through time in response to societal needs and the social and political structure in which nursing has existed.
- The base for nursing practice and nursing education as we currently know it was established by Florence Nightingale, who positively influenced health care standards, nursing practice, nursing education, and women's rights.
- Nursing education in North America has changed from service-oriented hospital training schools to educational programs primarily offered in colleges and universities.
- The roles, functions, and professional status of nursing have been defined and described by ICN, ANA, and CNA. In all definitions, the central focus of nursing is the person receiving the care.

■ Nursing is an emerging profession and discipline. It is a practice that applies knowledge through specialized skills, upholds standards developed by and for the profession, develops theories and conducts research, and uses the nursing process to give individualized and holistic care.

CRITICAL THINKING ACTIVITIES

1. Select a major figure in the history of nursing and give a report, verbally and/or in writing, on the influence of that person on past or current nursing practice.
2. Select a nurse in your local geographical area who has made a contribution to nursing. Invite him or her to attend a class and discuss some of his or her experiences, relating observed changes in nursing and forecasted trends.
3. Discuss potential challenges for the profession of nursing in the future.

BIBLIOGRAPHY

American Nurses Association. (1965). A position paper. New York: American Nurses Association Committee on Education.

Cooke, H. (1990). An introduction to the social history of nursing. *British Journal of Sociology, 41,* 593.

Curtin, L. L. (1990). Designing new roles: Nursing in the '90s and beyond. *Nursing Management, 21*(2), 7–8.

Deloughery, G. (1995). *Issues and trends in nursing.* St. Louis: Mosby.

Diers, D. (1990). The art and craft of nursing. *American Journal of Nursing, 90*(1), 65–66.

Dietz, L. D., & Lehozky, A. R. (1993). *History and modern nursing* (2nd ed.). Philadelphia: F. A. Davis Company.

Donahue, M. (1990). The past in the present. *Journal of Professional Nursing, 6,* 9.

Donahue, M. (1996). *Nursing, the finest art: An illustrated history* (2nd ed.). St. Louis: Mosby.

Jameson, E. M. (1968). *Trends in nursing history* (6th ed.). Philadelphia: W. B. Saunders.

Kalisch & Kalisch. (1995). *The advance of American nursing* (3rd ed.). Philadelphia: Lippincott.

Kenny, E. (1986). An LP looks at the developing LP role. *Issues, 7*(2), 6.

Macrae, J. (1995). Nightingale's spiritual philosophy and its significance for modern nursing. *Image: Journal of Nursing Scholarship, 27*(1), 8–10.

Mason, D. J., & Lewitt, J. K. (1995). The revolution in health-care: What's your readiness quotient? *American Journal of Nursing, 95*(6), 50–54.

Mitchell, P. R., & Grippando, G. M. (1993). *Nursing perspectives and issues* (5th ed.). New York: Delmar.

Mosby's medical, nursing and allied health dictionary (4th ed.). (1994). St. Louis: Mosby.

Woodham, S. G. (1981). *Florence Nightingale.* New York: McGraw-Hill.

INTERNET RESOURCES

American Association for the History of Nursing
http://www.aahn.org
American Nurses Association
http://www.nursingworld.org
Florence Nightingale Museum
http://www.florence-nightingale.co.uk
National League for Nursing Committee on Accreditation
http://www.accrediting-comm-nlnac.org
National Student Nurses Association
http://www.nsna.org
Nursing Net
http://www.nursingnet.org

CHAPTER 2

Health Care Delivery Systems

OVERVIEW

This chapter introduces concepts such as community-based health care, collaborative care, the financial aspects, and selected trends and issues affecting the health care system. This material discusses continuity of care as patients move among health care settings.

OBJECTIVES

Upon completion of this chapter, the reader should be able to:

- Compare and contrast the different community-based settings in which health care is provided.
- Describe community-based health care agencies and services.
- Discuss the elements of managed care, case management, and primary health care.
- Discuss various methods of financing health care in the United States.
- Discuss trends and issues affecting health care delivery.
- Describe special considerations unique to home care management.

KEY TERMS

Ambulatory care	Medicaid
Case management	Medicare
Community-based health care	Outpatient
Consumer	Preferred provider organization
Diagnostic-related groups	Primary health care
Health maintenance organization	Public health agencies
Inpatient	Public Health Service
Long-term care	Rehabilitation centers
Managed care	Voluntary agencies

INTRODUCTION

Everyone is concerned about health care. Costs seem to be rising exponentially and no one wants to see children, senior citizens, or others go without adequate care. Yet the twin goals of cost containment and universal access to services often seem unattainable. The traditional hospital delivered health care does not seem capable of meeting these social goals. New settings and new financial models will need to be developed.

This chapter focuses on the various types of health care settings, including the home, acute care hospitals, and primary care and ambulatory care centers, and specialized care centers. Long-term care and hospice services will be discussed. The frameworks for care include a presentation on managed care and case management. The financial aspects of health care focus on federally funded health care programs, group plans, and health maintenance organizations. Finally, the uniqueness of home care management is discussed and a presentation on the challenges in financial and resource management is included.

HEALTH CARE SETTINGS

It is estimated that there are over 7,000 hospitals, 4,000 community health agencies, and 25,000 long-term care facilities in the United States. When one considers that only patients who require complex surgery, are acutely ill or seriously injured, or are having babies are hospitalized, it is clear that many health care services are provided in settings outside the hospital. Consideration of the patient's needs for health restoration and health promotion throughout the life span make nursing provided within a community-based framework essential.

Community-Based Health Care

Community-based health care is care that is provided to people who live within a defined geographic region or have common needs. It is holistic, considering all dimensions of the individual in both health and illness. Community-based health care is designed to meet needs of people as they move between and among health care settings.

Community-based health care is provided within many different types of settings. Services are provided in clinics, hospitals, homes, schools, and day-care centers for children and older people. Other settings include crisis intervention centers, mental health centers, drug and alcohol rehabilitation programs, store-front clinics, and churches. These centers provide a variety of services. Some community-based agencies provide immunizations for infants and children; screenings for sexually transmitted diseases (STDs) or tuberculosis; and verification of need and voucher distribution for milk and food for women and children with low incomes through the Women, Infants, and Children (WIC) program. Community-based health care may also focus on special needs, such as older adult or terminally ill patients. Nurses are involved in caring for patients and families in all of these settings and more.

People requiring care are often categorized as either inpatients or outpatients. When people enter a health care setting, such as a hospital and stay for more than 24 hours, they are said to be **inpatients**. In an effort to reduce costs as well as quickly return patients to their homes and families, there has been a proliferation of services offered for the **outpatient**—the person who requires health care services but does not need to stay in an institution for those services. Individuals who do not require inpatient care receive treatment, care, and education and are then sent home. Examples of services provided on an outpatient basis include surgical procedures, diagnostic tests, medications, physical therapy, counseling, and health education. These services are rapidly expanding and are now commonly provided by hospitals, health care providers' offices, ambulatory care centers, and clinics. Many hospitals now maintain short-stay units, where patients having diagnostic tests or surgery enter the hospital, have the procedure, and then return to the hospital room for a brief (from 1 to 6 hours) recovery period before going home.

Hospitals: Acute Care Settings

When most people hear "health care," they think of hospitals. This is not surprising. Hospitals are the traditional setting for care. People who were too ill to care for themselves at home, who were severely injured, who required surgery or complicated treatments, or who were having babies were typically admitted to the hospital. They received treatment and were not discharged until they were fully recovered or used all of the services available within the hospital. This is changing. As a result of federal regulations and other health care reimbursement policies, patients are returning home earlier and earlier. Hospitals now focus more often on the acute needs of the patient.

Hospital size ranges from as few as twenty beds to large medical centers with hundreds of beds. Various services are provided, depending on the size and location of the hospital. Most hospitals provide emergency care, inpatient care, surgery, diagnostic tests, and patient education. Other services provided within the hospital setting might include intensive care units, obstetrical care, social services, outpatient clinics and surgery, educational programs, and long-term skilled nursing facilities. Hospitals may provide care for all types of illnesses and trauma, or may specialize. Specialty hospitals, or special units in general hospitals, meet the varied needs of patients, including children, patients needing rehabilitation, patients requiring psychiatric care, and patients with severe burns.

Hospitals are classified as public or private and as for-profit or not-for-profit. Public hospitals, which are not-for-profit institutions, are financed and operated by local, state, or national agencies. Many patients admitted to a public hospital do not have health insurance, and services are provided at no cost or at little cost to the patient. The cost is covered by taxes or public funds. Private hospitals may be for-profit or not-for-profit and are operated by communities, churches, businesses or corporations, and charitable organizations. Many patients cared for in private hospitals have some type of personal health insurance or health care plan.

Canadian hospitals receive funding from federal and provincial sources. Patients have basic health insurance specific to the province in which they reside. In addition, some patients have private health

ASK YOURSELF

If you were invited to participate on the project of developing basic essential health care services to which all persons would have access, what services would you include? Would you include community-based health care services? How would you provide for funding?

insurance plans or health plans through employment that provide extended coverage and additional benefits.

Although trends are changing, hospitals still employ more nurses than any other type of facility. Nurses employed in the hospital setting have many roles. Although many nurses are direct care providers, other roles include manager of other members of the health care team that provides patient care, administrator, nurse practitioner, clinical nurse specialist, patient educator, in-service educator, and researcher. The current emphasis on cost containment and restructuring has made and will continue to make changes in where and how nurses work.

Home Health Care

Home care is one of the most rapidly growing areas in the health care system. Caring for patients may be provided in their homes through community health departments, visiting nurses' associations, hospital-based case managers, and home health agencies. These agencies provide many different health-related services, including skilled nursing assessment, teaching and support of patients and family members, and direct care for patients (Figure 2–1 and Table 2–1).

Nurses who work in this type of setting make assessments and provide physical care, administer medications, teach, and support family members. They also collaborate with other health care providers such as physicians, physical therapists (PTs), occupational therapists, and respiratory therapists (RTs) to plan and provide patient care.

Primary Care Centers

Primary health care services are provided by physicians in their offices through diagnosis and treatment of minor illnesses, minor surgical

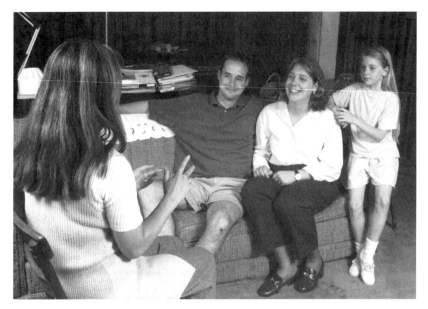

FIGURE 2–1 It is important not to overload a family with too much information all at one time.

procedures, obstetric care, well-child care, counseling and referrals. Many offices contain laboratory and x-ray facilities. Although some physicians are general practitioners who treat all types of illnesses, many physicians now specialize in one type of illness or surgery.

TABLE 2–1
Factors Influencing the Importance of Home Health Care

The importance of home health care is evidenced by several factors, including the following:

- The prospective payment system of reimbursement (DRGs), which encourages early discharge from the hospital, has created a new, acutely ill population that needs skilled care at home.
- There are increasing numbers of older people living longer with multiple chronic illnesses who are not institutionalized.
- With more sophisticated technology, people can be kept alive and relatively comfortable in their own homes.
- Health care consumers demand that services be humane and that provisions be made for a dignified death at home.

A nurse in a physician's office makes health assessments, performs technical skills, assists the physician, and provides health education. Some offices include a nurse practitioner or clinical nurse specialist who works collaboratively with the physician to make assessments and care for patients who require health maintenance or health promotion activities. Nurse practitioners are also establishing offices and clinics to provide primary care and treatment to patients and only refer complex health problems to a physician.

Ambulatory Care Centers

Ambulatory care centers and clinics may be located in hospitals. They may also be provided as a freestanding service by a group of physicians who work together, or may be by a nurse practitioner. Ambulatory care centers and clinics are often located in areas that are convenient for people. It is not uncommon to find a center in a shopping mall or other community setting. Many ambulatory care centers and clinics offer walk-in services so that appointments are unnecessary. Stressing convenience, they are also open at times other than traditional office hours. Nurses in these centers and clinics provide technical skills (such as administering medications), determine the priority of care needs and patients, and educate patients about all aspects of care. A special type of ambulatory care center is an urgent care center that provides walk-in emergency care services. Ambulatory surgical centers are another form of ambulatory care center.

Specialized Care Centers

Specialized care centers provide services for a special population or group. They are usually located in easily accessible locations within a community.

Day-Care Centers

Day-care centers have a variety of purposes. Some centers provide care for infants and children who are healthy but need attention and super-vision while parents work. Often these centers also care for children with minor illnesses. Elder-care centers and senior citizen centers provide a place for older adults to socialize and to receive care while family members work. Some day-care centers provide health-related services and care to people who do not necessarily need to be in a health care institution but cannot be at home alone. These include centers for older patients requiring physical rehabilitation; patients with special needs (e.g., cerebral palsy); patients who are in drug and alcohol programs; and patients requiring mental health services. Nurses who work in day-care centers administer medications and treatments, conduct health screenings, teach, and counsel.

Mental Health Centers

Mental health centers may be associated with a hospital or they may provide services as an independent agency. The services provided are often crisis centered. Suicide hotlines are an excellent example of a crisis-related mental health center. Others involve long-term counseling. Long-term facilities provide outpatient care through a variety of interventions, including individual and group counseling, prescription of medications, and assistance with independent living. Crisis intervention centers, by contrast, typically provide 24-hour services and hotlines for people who are suicidal who are abusing drugs or alcohol, and who require psychologic or psychiatric counseling. These crisis-related centers also provide information and services for victims of rape and abuse. Nurses who work in mental health centers must have strong communication and counseling skills, and must be thoroughly familiar with community resources specific to the needs of patients being served.

Rural Health Centers

Rural health centers are often located in geographically remote areas. These centers seek to address the unique needs of rural areas with a low economic base and few health care providers. Many rural health centers are run by nurse practitioners, who serve as the patient's primary health provider for the care of minor acute illnesses as well as chronic illness care. Patients who are seriously ill or injured are given emergency care and transferred to the nearest large hospital. Nurses who practice independently do so in collaboration with a physician who approves protocols for care. Many rural hospitals, physicians, and nurse practitioners now have immediate access to information about diagnosis and treatment of illness through telecommunications and computers.

Schools

Although schools are not traditionally considered to be a health care setting, school nurses are often the major source of health assessment, health education, and emergency care for the nation's children. The role of the school nurse reflects changes in society itself. Children in schools today are from many different racial and ethnic groups. They have varying socioeconomic backgrounds, and many have more complex disabilities requiring expert knowledge and skills for management during school hours. School nurses provide a great number of different services, including maintaining immunization records, providing emergency care for physical and mental illnesses, administering prescribed medications, conducting routine health screenings (such as those for vision, hearing, and scoliosis), and providing information about health.

Industry

Many large industries have their own ambulatory care clinic, staffed primarily by nurses. Occupational health nurses practicing in industrial clinics focus on preventing work-related injury and illness. They conduct health assessments, encourage wellness (such as stopping smoking, eating sensibly, and exercising regularly), care for minor injuries and illnesses, and make referrals for more serious health problems.

Homeless Shelters

Homeless shelters are usually living units (such as an apartment building or home) that provide housing for people who do not have regular shelter. The homeless are at increased risk for illness or injury for many reasons. They face threats such as exposure to the elements, violence, drug and alcohol addiction, poor nutrition, poor hygiene, and overcrowding. Nurses who provide health care services to the homeless must be sensitive, nonjudgmental, and caring. The type of service provided by nurses may include immunizing children, teaching pregnant women, treating infections and illnesses, referring for diagnosis of sexually transmitted diseases, and providing information about maintaining health.

Rehabilitation Centers

Rehabilitation centers specialize in services for patients requiring physical or emotional rehabilitation and for treatment of any type of drug dependency. The centers may be freestanding or may be associated with a hospital. The goal is to return patients to optimal health and to the community as productive members of society. Centers that focus on rehabilitation use a health care team composed of different members such as physicians, nurses, PTs, OTs, and counselors. The role of the nurse includes direct care, teaching, and counseling. The practice of rehabilitation nursing is based on a philosophy of encouraging independent self-care within the patient's capabilities.

Long-Term Care Facilities

Those who are physically or mentally unable to care for themselves independently receive care in a **long-term care** facility. The care may extend for periods ranging from days to years. Settings that provide long-term care are usually independent facilities, but may also be associated with a hospital. Examples of long-term care facilities include: nursing homes, retirement centers, and residential institutions for mentally and developmentally or physically disabled patients of all ages.

Long-term care facilities proliferated for two main reasons. First, hospitals are discharging patients earlier in their recovery period. These recovering people often require care that is beyond the scope of home care. This group of patients receives transitional, subacute care in a long-term facility. Second, the number of older adults is increasing more rapidly than any other age group. Many of these older adults do not have any caregivers. As a result they are no longer able to carry out ordinary daily activities independently. Others simply do not want to continue maintaining a home.

Although long-term care facilities—especially nursing homes—often had a negative image, much has changed in recent years. Most nursing homes now focus on maintaining both patient function and independence, with concern for the living environment as well as the health care provided. Concern for the happiness as well as the health of nursing home residents has led to surroundings that include plants and animals as part of the home. Many of the overall improvements in long-term care came about as a result of the 1987 Omnibus Budget Reconciliation Act (OBRA); as part of that act, legislation was passed to maintain standards of quality assurance in the nursing home industry.

Because residents entering long-term care facilities require so many levels of care, it is difficult to generalize about services provided. In some instances, an older adult may choose to move into a retirement center that provides health care services only when needed. Other people who enter a nursing home may require complete care for as long as they live. Those individuals entering convalescent centers only remain until they are considered recovered. The nurse's role in a long-term care facility may be as a provider of direct care, supervisor, administrator, or teacher. Because most patients are older, increasing numbers of gerontology nurse specialists are contributing their knowledge and expertise to the care of these patients. Almost all long-term care facilities require that skilled nursing care be available at all times. The care given to patients can only be performed by or under the direct supervision of a licensed nurse.

Hospice Services

Hospices are special services available to terminally ill individuals and their families. The provider may be public or private and may offer both inpatient and home care. These agencies are committed to maintaining both quality of life and dignity for the dying person. An environment that encourages open communication, symptom management, and comfort measures for the patient is emphasized. Many also offer support to the family during and after death of the patient. Many hospice agencies are developed and supervised by nurses but use trained volunteers to supply much needed assistance. These volunteers provide emotional and physical support, and assist with transportation and household care. It is not uncommon for these unpaid aides to serve as liaison between the patient and health care providers, and provide short-term respite care for family members.

HEALTH CARE AGENCIES

Many different types of agencies provide health care services within a community. Those discussed here are voluntary agencies, religious agencies, and government agencies.

Voluntary Agencies

Community agencies are often not-for-profit organizations. These groups are financed by private donations, grants, or fundraisers (although some may charge minimal fees). An example of a volunteer agency is Meals on Wheels, which supplies meals, transportation services, and shopping or housecleaning services for senior citizens, the disabled, and other homebound people. Other examples include the Heart Association and the Lung Association. Physicians and nurses are often active members of these organizations and provide health screenings and educational programs.

Voluntary agencies also provide the setting for support groups. These bodies are designed to provide education and a support for patients who wish to adjust to new or existing health problems. Members of support groups typically experienced the same type of problem at one time. By sharing problems, members learn to solve problems and cope with a stressful or crisis situation (Table 2–2).

TABLE 2–2

Examples of Support Groups

Alcoholics Anonymous, an international organization for recovering alcoholics. The purpose of the support group is to help individuals stop drinking and remain sober. Meetings are held in an accessible community location such as a church or hospital.

Cancer support groups, which focus on support and solving problems experienced by people diagnosed with cancer. Many cancer support group meetings are held at a hospital.

Reach to Recovery is a support group for women who have had a breast removed due to cancer or have had breast surgery, including breast reconstruction. Among other activities, members visit women prior to surgery, teach exercises to prevent muscle atrophy, and provide information about prostheses and clothing.

Religious Agencies

Parish nursing is an area of community-based nursing practice that emphasizes holistic health care, health promotion, and disease prevention activities. Parish nursing is based on the belief that health promotion means reaching people before they become sick. Activities are often volunteer affairs and they are frequently based within a church, synagogue, or mosque. Parish nurses function as health educators, resource and referral persons, and facilitators of lay volunteer and support groups. These nurses reach out to vulnerable populations—the elderly, single parents, and children.

Government Agencies

National, state/provincial, and local governments support a great number of health care bodies and organizations. City taxes, for instance, support city hospitals and public health clinics. States or provinces support state mental health hospitals and other facilities and programs. National governments also assume an active role in health care. In many countries tax revenue is used to finance national health and welfare programs such as Canada's Department of Health and Welfare.

Veterans Administration

Veterans Administration (VA) hospitals and military hospitals all come under the umbrella of government-supported and government-operated health care. VA hospitals provide health care services to veterans, and military hospitals provide care to members of the armed forces and their immediate families.

Public Health Service

The **Public Health Service** (PHS) is a federal health agency that falls under the direction of the U.S. Department of Health and Human Services. A similar health service is provided by the Department of Health and Welfare in Canada. PHS is a multifaceted program that covers a wide range of services. It is the medical branch of the U.S. Coast Guard and the principal source of Native American health care through the Indian Health Services. The amount of direct patient care provided by PHS is more limited than in the past. PHS also supplies funds to health centers that provide care to migrant workers and to community agencies that supply health care to the poor or uninsured. The principal budget of PHS goes to grant programs for poor and uninsured individuals.

Additionally, the Centers for Disease Control and Prevention (CDC) and the National Institutes of Health (NIH) are both part of PHS. CDC focuses on the epidemiology, prevention, control, and treatment of communicable diseases such as STDs. NIH is engaged in various health research activities.

PHS also supplies health care professionals (e.g., nurses, physicians, dentists, and pharmacists) to the U.S. Department of Justice to provide care in federal prisons. The service is also involved to varying degrees in drug and alcohol abuse and mental health programs within the state. PHS activities vary from area to area. In most cases, they focus on community needs and attempt to meet those needs whenever possible.

The types of government health care services and agencies available in Canada are similar to those in the United States. The major difference between the two systems is the way that health care is financed. The Canadian health care system is financed by health care plans within each province. These plans cover all Canadian residents for most of their necessary hospital care and physicians' fees. These provincial health insurance plans are financed by federal and provincial taxes, employers, or personal policies.

Public Health Agencies

Public health agencies are local, state or provincial, or federal agencies that provide public health services to members of various sizes of communities (i.e., local, county, provincial, state, or federal). Public health departments are usually funded by taxes and often have administrators who are elected or appointed. Local agencies provide services and programs to prevent illness and promote health, such as tuberculosis screening, immunizations, and sexually transmitted disease screening. Public health agencies work collaboratively with state and local departments to ensure health through activities such as inspections of restaurants and water supplies. They also provide educational programs and may provide direct care services for low-income people or people living in rural, isolated areas. Nurses who practice in public health agencies focus on prenatal care, well-child care, screening programs, education, and outreach into the community.

FRAMEWORKS FOR CARE

There are different methods for ensuring continuity of care and cost-effective care as a patient moves through the health care system. These methods include managed care systems, case management, and primary health care.

Managed Care Systems

Managed care is an organized system of health care that influences the selection and use of high-quality and cost-effective health care services for a population. The care of an individual is carefully planned and monitored from the initial contact to discharge from a health care episode. Planning and monitoring activities are conducted to ensure that standards are followed and costs are minimized. More and more, health maintenance organizations (HMOs) and insurance companies are changing to managed care systems. A form of managed care was even proposed as a national health care plan.

Case Management

In the past eight to nine years, nursing case management emerged as an important method of coordinating care, controlling costs, and improving access to health care (Figure 2–2).

Case management is a process of coordinating an individual patient's health care for the purpose of maximizing positive outcomes and containing costs. Although there are several different forms of case management, all focus on enhancing continuity of care and effectively using health care resources. The primary objective in many case management systems is to identify specific protocols and timetables for

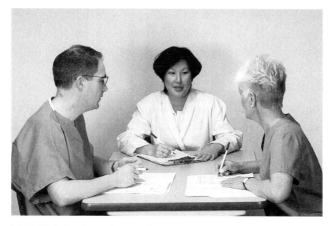

FIGURE 2-2 Through consultation and exchange of information, nurses demonstrate their roles as autonomous professionals. How important are the qualities of empowerment and autonomy to your own career?

care and treatment in a format called a critical pathway. Critical pathways incorporate independent and collaborative nursing interventions to reach desired patient outcomes within a specific time frame.

The nurse case manager is responsible for the goals and may follow the patient from diagnosis of an illness to hospitalization and then back to home care. During the health care episode, the nurse case manager is responsible for managing the patient's interactions with the entire health care system (Table 2–3).

TABLE 2-3

Nurse Case Manager Functions

- Coordinating care within a managed care system to effectively meet consumer health care needs and organization cost-containment needs
- Working with patients within a health insurance system to approve high-cost items such as diagnostic tests and hospital admission
- Working within a hospital system to make admission procedures more timely, and to coordinate services while the patient is hospitalized
- Establishing wellness programs in corporations
- Establishing a private practice to focus on a specific group of patients, such as the older adult

Nurses who are case managers do not give direct patient care; rather they coordinate the care provided by others. In this role, nurse case managers have increased autonomy and power within the health care system.

Clinical Pathways

An important element of resource management, especially in the health care setting, is the incorporation of practice protocols, case management, and clinical pathways into the care planning of a given patient population. It is important to note that clinical pathways or care protocols have financial implications, because they dictate the types and amounts of care given.

Clinical pathways are a set of clinical tools that organize, sequence, and time the major interventions of the nursing staff and physicians for a particular case type, condition, diagnostic category, or nursing diagnosis. Additionally, the pathways may also describe an institution's collective standard of practice. They can provide a direction and predictability to patient care and to the caregivers interacting in the clinical case. The Agency for Healthcare Policy and Research (AHCPR), funded by the Department of Health and Human Services (DHHS), has done a tremendous amount of research in the development of nationally accepted protocols for care of certain disease conditions. These protocols may be used in the development of individual institutional care practices or clinical paths as the foundation for different clinicians from the various health professions to begin the discussion of standardization of the many facets of health care. With increased and improved standardization, outcome of care can be studied and scrutinized to determine the practices that will best lead to positive outcomes for all parties involved.

As a direct link to the controlling of costs, clinical paths are also integral to improving care processes, because variances gleaned from clinical path implementation should be reviewed and analyzed to improve the care process. Clinical paths are not for all patients or conditions and need to be adjusted for complexity and acuity of patients. Paths are a tool in the arsenal of health care providers to standardize, control, and ultimately improve care through scrutiny of measured outcomes.

Diagnostic-Related Groups

Another resource set that is useful to achieve patient care outcomes is **diagnostic-related groups**. It is important to understand the complexities of the resources needed and nurses must be aware of the fiscal constraints placed on operations for the proper use of limited resources. Diagnostic-related groups is a classification system that was developed in the 1980s and adopted by the Health Care Financing Administration (HCFA) to control the cost of health care to its Medicare beneficiaries by assigning a cost by diagnostic category to include all services provided.

Primary Health Care

Primary health care was originally conceptualized in 1978 by the World Health Organization (WHO) and the United Nations International Children's Emergency Fund (UNICEF). The concept was developed based on decreases in illness and death in member countries that were achieved by simple, local, inexpensive solutions to health problems especially when combined with economic and social development. Further discussion led to the Alma-Ata declaration, which focused on a global health strategy called primary health care. This emphasized essential health care based on practical, scientifically sound, and socially acceptable methods and technology. It was to be made universally accessible to individuals and families in the community through their full participation and at a cost the community can afford. Finally, it should bring health care as close as possible to where people live and work.

Primary health care differs from primary care. Primary care is the delivery of health care services, including the initial contact and ongoing care. Included in primary care is the responsibility for referral to other providers based on patient needs. Both physicians and nurse practitioners provide primary care, which has an individual patient, provider-directed focus. In contrast, primary health care has a community-based philosophical base that emphasizes universal access and affordability of health care, health of the population, and consumer involvement. However, it is important to remember that primary care, as well as case management, can be practiced within a primary health care philosophy.

Collaborative Care

No matter what the type of setting or framework for care, the nurse works with a variety of professionals as patient care is planned, provided, and evaluated. For example, the nurse may request a consultation with a dietitian for a patient who is not eating well or for another who needs to lose weight. After the dietitian talks with the patient and determines a plan of care, the nurse can reinforce the plan and evaluate its effectiveness. Collaboration between and among nurses is also an essential part of holistic patient care. The primary goal of each member of the health care team is to promote wellness and restore health. Included in this section is a discussion of each member of the health care team (other than nurses) with whom you will be working most often.

Physician

The physician is primarily responsible for the diagnosis and the medical or surgical treatment of an illness. Physicians are granted the authority to admit patients to health care settings by a health care agency or institution. They are also permitted to practice care within the setting through such actions as writing orders, interpreting the results of laboratory and diagnostic tests, performing procedures and surgery, and working collaboratively with other professionals. Individuals become physicians after extensive education and clinical practice and by passing a licensing examination. Depending on the curriculum completed, a physician may graduate from a medical school and become a Doctor of Medicine (MD) or may graduate from a college of osteopathy and become a Doctor of Osteopathy (DO). Both the MD and DO have almost exactly the same type of education and areas of practice, but osteopathic medicine emphasizes the study of mechanical changes in tissues as a cause of illness and treatment that involves manipulation of body structures. Physicians may choose to be general practitioners, or may choose to specialize in the treatment of one type of illness (such as a cardiologist) or a specific type of surgery (such as an orthopedic surgeon).

 ASK YOURSELF

In your community, are any health care services not being delivered by physicians? What segments of the population are being served? Where are these services being delivered? In clinics, private practice offices, or hospitals?

Physician's Assistant (PA)

A PA has completed specific courses of study as preparation for providing support to the physician and does take a licensing examination. The PA's responsibilities usually depend on the physician supervising the activities, and might include conducting physical examinations and suturing lacerations. In most states, a nurse is not legally bound to follow a PA's orders unless they are cosigned by a physician. This is an important aspect to investigate if PAs are employed by a prospective employer.

Physical Therapist (PT)

A PT works to restore function or prevent further disability in a patient after an injury or illness. The PT uses various techniques to treat patients, including massage, heat, cold, water, sonar waves, exercises, and electrical stimulation. Most PTs are also educated in the use of psychologic strategies to motivate patients.

Respiratory Therapist (RT)

An RT has been trained in techniques that improve pulmonary function and oxygenation. RTs may also be responsible for administering a variety of tests that measure lung functioning and for educating the patient on the use of various devices and machines prescribed by the physician.

Occupational Therapist (OT)

An OT assists the physically challenged patient to adapt to limitations. The OT uses a variety of adaptive devices and strategies to aid a patient in carrying out activities of daily living.

Speech Therapist

A speech therapist is trained to help hearing-impaired patients speak more clearly, to assist a patient who has had a stroke to relearn how to speak, and to correct or modify a variety of speech disturbances in children and adults. Speech therapists also diagnose and treat swallowing problems in patients who have had a head injury or a stroke.

Dietitian

Generally, a registered dietitian (RD) is responsible for managing and planning the dietary needs of patients. The RD is knowledgeable about all aspects of nutrition and its effects on the body. An RD can adapt specialized diets for the individual needs of patients, counsel and educate individual patients, and supervise the dietary services of the entire facility.

Pharmacist

A pharmacist is licensed to formulate and dispense medications. The pharmacist is also responsible for keeping a running file of all patient medications and for informing the physician when a potential or actual medication error in prescribing has occurred or when prescribed drugs may interact adversely. The pharmacist is an excellent resource for both patients and nurses for any information related to medications.

Social Worker

A social worker counsels patients and family members and also informs them of and refers them to various community resources. The role of the social worker encompasses many activities, such as counseling, reporting suspected drug addiction or abuse, assisting with decisions about life-sustaining treatments, adopting children, and placing patients in long-term care facilities.

Spiritual Counselor

Most agencies employ a chaplain, rabbi, or other religious figure to give spiritual support and guidance to patients and their families. The advisor may also refer a patient to a priest, minister, or rabbi of the patient's own religious denomination. Many hospitals and health care agencies have collaborative relationships with the religious bodies in the local community and the pastors, pastoral assistants, deacons, and other designated representatives of the church are welcome and encouraged to visit their members who are hospitalized or reside in long-term care facilities. These persons will administer certain specific religious rites, including communion, prayer, anointing, and baptisms. Nurses are frequently asked to assist the patient in preparing for religious rites; however, it is important to respect the patient's wishes regarding privacy during the religious rites and activities.

FINANCIAL ASPECTS OF HEALTH CARE

Health care is very expensive, with costs continuing to increase. Few citizens can afford to pay for health care from personal resources. The costs of health care are often covered by the federal government and private organizations through federally funded programs, prepaid plans, and private insurance.

Federally Funded Programs

The federally funded health care programs are primarily through Medicare and Medicaid. The history of federally funded health care, legislated by the federal government, is summarized as follows:

In 1965 **Medicare** amendments to the Social Security Act established national and state health insurance programs for the elderly under Title 18. Within a decade, almost all citizens over the age of 65 held Medicare insurance for hospital care, extended care, and home health care.

In the same year, **Medicaid** was established under Title 19 of the Social Security Act. This program is a federally funded public assistance program for people with low incomes.

In 1972, Medicare coverage was increased to include permanently disabled workers and their dependents if they also qualified for Social Security benefits.

In 1983, Medicare converted to a prospective payment plan called diagnosis-related groups (DRGs). This plan pays the hospital a predetermined, fixed amount that is determined by the medical diagnosis or specific procedure rather than by the actual cost of hospitalization and care. DRGs were implemented by the federal government in an effort to control rising health care costs. The plan pays only the amount of money preassigned to a diagnosis (e.g., an appendectomy); if the cost for hospitalization is greater than that assigned, the hospital must absorb the additional cost. However, if costs are less than those assigned, the hospital makes a profit. In 1988, Medicare was again expanded to include catastrophic care costs and expensive medications.

People who receive Medicare pay both a deductible cost and a monthly premium for full insurance coverage. Part A of Medicare, which pays most inpatient hospital costs, is paid by the federal government. Part B of Medicare, which is voluntary, is paid by monthly premiums; it covers most outpatient costs for physician visits, medications, and home health services. The full cost of some services is not covered by Medicare; it is recommended that patients subscribe to supplemental insurance policies offered by private insurance companies. Also, because Medicare is federally funded, benefits may change annually according to decisions made concerning the federal budget.

Current budgetary considerations are forcing state and federal agencies to trim Medicaid expenditures. The rapid growth of an aging population and an increase in the number of poor people, many of whom are women and children, are draining the Medicaid budget. For survival, Medicaid programs are implementing reforms such as reduced benefits, or are placing patients into managed care programs.

Group Plans

Group plans for financing health care in the United States include health maintenance organizations (HMOs), preferred provider organizations (PPOs), and private insurance. Enrollment in these plans is voluntary. An individual pays a fixed rate on either a monthly or annual plan and, in turn, receives financial coverage for all the health care necessary to maintain wellness and treat illness. Because group plans such as HMOs and PPOs assume the financial loss or gain of the health care services used by their clients, they encourage preventive health care to avoid the higher costs of illness and hospitalization. For the same reason, these plans carefully monitor the quality and quantity of the health care delivered to clients. They also place limitations on the use of high-cost procedures and require certain guidelines to be followed when a higher-cost procedure is recommended by a physician. Some people do not like these plans because they use a selective contracting approach, mandating subscriber use of specific institutions and health care providers. Some consumers dislike the lack of control they have in making decisions relating to personal or family health.

Health Maintenance Organizations

Health maintenance organizations (HMOs) are prepaid group health care plans that allow enrollees to receive all the medical services they require through a group of affiliated providers. There are often no additional out-of-pocket costs, or the enrollees may pay only a small fee, called a copay. An HMO may employ all its providers (including physicians) or may be formed by a group of physicians in alliance who provide care as independent practitioners (an independent practice association or IPA). In most HMO structures, the patient does not have a choice about health care providers, and receives all services from physicians associated with or who are part of the HMO. HMOs are becoming more popular, especially with larger employers, because they do support the concept of managed care.

Preferred Provider Organizations

Preferred provider organizations (PPOs) allow a third-party payer (such as a health insurance company) to contract with a group of health care providers to provide services at a lower fee in return for prompt payment and a guaranteed volume of patients and services. However, patients have more choices: Although they are encouraged to use specific providers, they may also seek care outside the panel without referral and pay additional out-of-pocket expenses. A form of this type of insurance plan is the preferred provider arrangement (PPA). In a PPA, the contract is made with an individual health care provider rather than with a group of providers. Similarly, a point-of-service (POS) plan encourages the use of specified physicians and services, but pays a portion of expenses if referrals are made to physicians outside the organization.

Private Insurance

Personal health care may be financed by private insurance; through large, nonprofit, tax-exempt organizations; or through smaller, private, for-profit insurance companies. To be insured, members pay monthly premiums either by themselves or in combination with their employer. These plans are called third-party payers because the insurance pays all or most of the cost of care. The premiums on private insurance plans tend to be higher than with HMOs, but the patient can choose the physician and services desired.

Long-Term Care Insurance

An interesting development in the health care insurance market is the growing interest in long-term care (LTC) insurance. In general, a minimal amount of LTC is paid for by private insurance. Most LTC (about 90 percent) is paid for by Medicaid and out-of-pocket spending. Medicare pays for a small percentage of LTC. The steady increase in the population of people aged 65 and older has become a major concern within the health care financing area.

Some commercial insurance companies offer LTC benefits. Promoters of LTC insurance have developed models of plans that would cover a variety of services such as nursing home care and home care as well as other services that would help prevent the institutionalization of older, debilitated, and chronically ill people. Adult day-care centers and respite care would also fall under these types of services and would be covered by benefits.

TRENDS AND ISSUES IN HEALTH CARE

Nurses need to be both personally and professionally aware of the major issues and trends that are shaping health care. The impact by public and private efforts to cope with rising health care costs, and the need to care for those without access to health care insurance, will be experienced by nurses as vital members of the health care team. Many nurses feel threatened by changes that they perceive as negative. Others embrace the challenges and seek to work within the system in order to guide change.

Focus on Wellness

Health awareness and the desire for personal involvement in one's own health care has strongly influenced the delivery of health care services in society. A consensus is emerging that it is better to remain healthy than it is to neglect one's health and then treat a resulting illness or injury. This belief has far-reaching influences on the way we live. Stress management programs, nutritional awareness, exercise and fitness programs, and anti-smoking and anti-drug campaigns are all examples of this trend. Equally important are measures such as promoting the wearing of seat belts, promoting automobile and airplane safety, controlling smog, controlling handguns, and eliminating hazardous wastes.

A public interest in self-care has evolved into a strong force in terms of the education and services provided by health care professionals. Consumers of health care are often better educated about health, prefer to control and make decisions about their own personal health, and want to be active participants in planning and implementing their own health care.

Consumer Movement

A **consumer** is someone who uses a commodity or service. Consumers of health care services are better educated today about the services they require and the services that are available. They are also concerned about access to services and the cost of those services. Consumers today question escalating costs and the proliferation and duplication of services. Patients as consumers are becoming actively involved in the administration of health care agencies and have developed standards for care, patient rights, and cost-containment measures as protection for patients when they enter a health care setting. On the other hand, the consumer movement has also led to an increase in malpractice lawsuits, resulting in high malpractice insurance rates (especially for physicians) and the necessity to carefully document care given. The increased paperwork often serves to take the nurse away from actual patient care.

Freedom of Choice

According to recent studies, consumer demand is pushing more insurance companies to consider offering coverage for alternative or complementary medicine. Services commonly covered include chiropractic and acupuncture. Other plans cover therapies such as massage, homeopathy, naturopathy, stress management, and traditional Chinese medicine.

Insurance companies and HMOs that offer alternative and complementary medical coverage usually work with physicians and nurses who also are alternative care providers or who include licensed acupuncturists, chiropractors, or other therapists in their medical group.

Cost Containment

The health care delivery system is experiencing a financial crisis. Health costs have increased dramatically, and some analysts believe that many cost-containment measures were implemented too late to effectively reverse the current upward swing in health costs. The actual short-term and long-term results of these cost-containment measures remain to be seen.

Historically, the health care system and the financial arrangements for paying for health care encouraged the use of expensive and sometimes inappropriate or ineffective health services. Many insurance plans paid for inpatient hospital care but not for ambulatory outpatient care. Therefore, to receive payment, patients were often hospitalized unnecessarily. Health care has also focused on the treatment of illnesses instead of on their prevention because preventive strategies often were not covered by a patient's health insurance policy. Third-party reimbursement effectively insulated patients from knowing the actual cost of their health care. Because the insurance company was responsible for paying the incurred bills, the patient was often bypassed in this process and seldom saw the bills for the care received.

Increased competition among hospitals further fueled the increase in health care costs. Technologically, amazing advances have been made, but as new machines and more advanced and expensive procedures are developed and used, patients' expectations of hospital resources will also increase. The media is constantly informing the public of new and innovative treatment modalities. Consumers expect these services to be available in "their" hospital. To attract patients, hospitals therefore feel compelled to invest huge sums of money in technologically advanced equipment. Supporters of cost-containment measures are encouraging hospitals to cooperate with one another and share resources rather than compete. Other efforts of cost containment include hospital restructuring and multiple hospitals joining together as one system.

Fragmentation of Care

Increased health care research has resulted in an upward spiral of technology and knowledge. In effect, this means that health care providers may no longer keep up with all of the advances made, so that specialization has become almost the rule rather than the exception. What does this mean for the patient?

A physician who is a general practitioner diagnoses and treats a variety of common health problems. However, a patient who requires diagnosis and treatment for a more complex problem is usually referred to a physician who is a specialist. For example, a patient with diabetes and a heart condition may be cared for by the family physician, a cardiologist, and an endocrinologist. The hospitalized patient not only comes in contact with many different health care providers (e.g., registered nurses, licensed practical/vocational nurses, nursing assistants, nurse specialists, physical therapists, dietitians, and students) but also is frequently seen by other physician specialists called in on consultation or to do surgery. It is no wonder that the patient becomes confused about care and treatments. This fragmentation of care can result in the loss of continuity of care, resulting in conflicting plans of care, too much or too little medication, and higher health care costs.

Changes in Patient Care Needs

The population of older adults, and particularly those over age 70, is the most rapidly growing segment of our population. As people age, there is an associated increase in chronic illnesses. This presents two problems. First, these patients require more health care in both in-patient and outpatient settings. As a result, hospitals are increasingly filled with older men and women who are in the acute or terminal stages of one or more chronic illnesses. Second, these patients need additional doctor's visits, more medications, and more health-related supplies; however, they often cannot afford to meet their health care needs, especially if they are on a fixed income. This problem is further compounded by a lack of transportation, a scarcity of family members or support systems, and a desire for independence that interferes with compliance with health care regimens. Many of these needs are also found in the growing number of people with AIDS and the homeless.

As current trends of wellness and prevention, consumerism, cost containment, and fragmentation of care continue into the new millennium, the delivery of health care will change as well. Governmental and private organizations will work to grapple successfully with an aging population, rural and urban poverty, and new technologies. Nurses need to be aware of these changes, and stand ready to influence them. Nursing professionals must continue to serve as the human component in the emerging health care delivery system.

KEY POINTS

- Community-based health care is care that is provided in all types of health care settings, is provided to people who live in a defined geographic area with common needs, is holistic, and is designed to meet the needs of the people as they move between and among health care settings.
- Community-based health care is provided in homes, hospitals, primary care centers, ambulatory care centers, specialized care centers, rehabilitation centers, long-term care facilities, hospices, and agencies. Nurses care for patients in all these settings and more.
- Health care services provided to patients in their homes include skilled nursing assessment, teaching and support of patients and family members, and direct care.
- Hospitals provide a wide variety of inpatient and outpatient services and are classified as either private or public, for-profit or not-for-profit. Care within the hospital setting is focused on the acute care needs of the patients.
- Primary health care services are provided in offices by physicians and nurse practitioners.
- Ambulatory care centers are often located in convenient areas, may offer walk-in services, and are open for a longer period than offices. Urgent-care centers provide emergency care services, and ambulatory surgical centers are sites for surgical procedures and care.
- Specialized care centers provide services for a specific population or group; they include day-care centers, mental health centers, rural health centers, schools, industry, and homeless shelters.
- Long-term centers provide care and support for physically and mentally challenged people of any age. Care, which may range from only a few days to years, includes transitional subacute care, intermediate and long-term care, and skilled care. Settings for

long-term care include hospitals, nursing homes, retirement centers, and residential institutions.

- Hospices provide special services for terminally ill patients and their families.
- Agencies that provide community-based health care services include voluntary agencies, religious agencies, and government agencies. Veterans hospitals, the Public Health Service, and public health agencies are also agencies that provide care and services to patients.
- Methods of ensuring continuity of care and cost-effective care include managed care systems, case management, and primary health care.
- Health care costs are financed through federally funded programs, group plans, and private health care insurance.
- Medicare is a federal health insurance program in the United States for people 65 years of age or older, for people with permanent kidney failure, and certain physically and mentally challenged individuals. Medicaid is a federally funded insurance program for people with low incomes.
- Current societal issues influencing health care delivery focus on wellness promotion, and include changes in patient care needs, cost containment, and consumer rights. Patients are better educated about health matters, prefer more control and more participation in decision making about personal health, and are becoming active participants in planning and implementing health care.

CRITICAL THINKING ACTIVITIES

1. Interview a nurse practitioner and discuss the required educational preparation, patients served, scope of practice, and challenges of advanced nursing practice.
2. Request a clinical assignment to work with a visiting nurse. Provide a report on the orientation to the clinical experience, the role and functions of the nurse in the field, collaborative efforts with other members of the health care team, time management skills, and documentation issues of the experience. Include input from an interview with the nurse with whom you are working.
3. Identify an acute care hospital in your local community. Find out about the types of services it provides, the type of ownership, the average length of stay, and the involvement in community activities. Analyze and discuss the contribution to health care in the community.

⇨ CASE STUDY

Mrs. Cameron is a 58-year-old hard-of-hearing woman who will have major surgery to replace a joint in her hip. She is married and employed as a school teacher. Her physician is concerned that she is about 25 pounds overweight. The case manager has met with the patient and it was determined that Mrs. Cameron does not participate in a personal program of wellness. A discharge planning conference is scheduled for this patient.

Design an agenda for the discharge planning session for Mrs. Cameron. Which hospital team members will be included as a part of the discharge planning conference? Will more than one planning conference be required? When will the patient and the family member (or caregiver) be included? Who are the key persons to be involved in assisting the patient in developing a personal program of wellness? How will the program of wellness be interdisciplined with the patient's postoperative rehabilitation program? Consider the need for inpatient rehabilitative care, a step-down unit, and outpatient care. Prepare a list of critical components of the Discharge Instruction Summary.

BIBLIOGRAPHY

American Public Health Association. (1990). *Healthy people 2000: National health promotion and disease prevention objectives.* Washington, DC: American Public Health Association.

Betts, V. (1995). Defining our future, dividing our resources. *American Nurse, 27*(3), 5.

Buerhaus, P. (1994). Managed competition and critical issues facing nurses. *Nursing and Healthcare, 15*(1), 22–26.

Dee-Kelly, P., Heller, S., & Sibley, M. (1994). Managed care: An opportunity for home care agencies. *Nursing Clinics of North America, 29*(3), 471–481.

Federa, R., & Camp, T. (1994). The changing managed care market. *Journal of Ambulatory Care Management, 17*(1), 1–7.

Feldstein, P. J. (1999). *Health care economics* (5th ed.). Albany, NY: Delmar Publishers.

Grace, H. K. (1997). Can medical costs be contained? In J. C. McCloskey & H. K. Grace (Eds.), *Current issues in nursing* (5th ed.). St. Louis: Mosby-Yearbook.

Hanah, K. J., Ball, M. J., & Edwards, M. J. A. (1994). *Introduction to nursing informatics.* New York: Springer-Verlag.

Hassett, M. M., & Farver, M. H. (1995). Information management in home care. In M. J. Ball, K. J. Hanah, S. K. Newbold, & J. V. Douglas (Eds.), *Nursing informatics: Where caring and technology meet* (2nd ed.). New York: Springer-Verlag.

Hicks, L. L., & Boles, K. E. (1997). Why health economics? In C. Harrington & C. L. Estes (Eds.), *Health policy and nursing: Crisis and reform in the U.S. health care delivery system* (2nd ed.). Boston: Jones & Bartlett.

King, J. (1993). Coalition building between public health nurses and parish nurses. *Journal of Nursing Administration, 23*(2), 27–31.

Sandhu, B. K., Duquette, A., & Kerouac, S. (1992). Care delivery modes. *Canadian Nurse, 88*(4), 18–20.

Shalala, D. (1993). Nursing & Society: The unfinished agenda for the 21st century. *Nursing & Healthcare, 14*(6), 289–291.

Uphold, C., & Graham, M. (1993). Schools as centers for collaborative services to families: A vision for change. *Nursing Outlook, 41*(5), 204–211.

Witek, J., & Hostage, J. (1994). Medicaid managed care: Problems and promises. *Journal of Ambulatory Care Management, 17*(1), 61–69.

Zerwekh, J., & Claborn, J. C. (1997). *Nursing today: Transitions and trends.* Philadelphia: W. B. Saunders.

INTERNET RESOURCES

Health hotlines
http://www.cdcnac.org/sis
Healthcare Internet Services
http://www.healthcareinternet.com
Patient advocacy numbers
http://www.infonet.welch.jhi.edu/advocacy.html
Support resources
http://www.cmhc.com/sxlist.htm

CHAPTER 3

Transcultural Nursing

➡ OVERVIEW

In today's health care arena, cultural sensitivity and skillfulness in interacting with people of various backgrounds is essential. A successful model for valuing diversity in practice is introduced in this chapter along with suggestions for creating an open, accepting environment. Cultural sensitivity is important. The way people work and interact with one another affects larger businesses and organizations, and ultimately, our own self worth and patient satisfaction. To enhance cultural awareness and sensitivity, relationships and interactions are discussed in terms of practical applications and general guidelines for patients from different backgrounds. The management of health care in today's changing marketplace is also emphasized in a presentation of cultural factors that may affect nursing care for several distinct ethnic and racial groups.

➡ OBJECTIVES

Upon completion of this chapter, the reader should be able to:

- Discuss the value of diversity in the health care setting.
- Outline four steps to create a workplace where diversity flourishes.
- Identify the do's and don'ts for managing a culturally diverse environment.
- Explore concepts of culturally sensitive patient care.
- Define four principles of practice that may be used to deliver sensitive care.
- Explain six phenomena evident in all cultural groups.
- Explore sensitive patient treatment approaches to patients of various cultures.

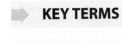

KEY TERMS

Cultural competence   Stereotyping

INTRODUCTION

Culture is shaped by values, beliefs, norms, and practices that are shared by members of the same group. Communications of specific cultures may be demonstrated through dress, style, language, and reaction to treatment modalities.

A major theme of transcultural nursing care is to focus on the caring practices of various cultures. Caring is a universal phenomenon, even though the forms and manifestations may vary among different groups. Caring practices are the protecting and assisting activities related to health and performed as part of a culture.

As practitioners, nurses allow culture to guide their thinking, doing, and being, as patterned expressions of who they are and how they practice. True change for the future may only be achieved if nurses understand the components of culture, its influence, and how it factors into the equation when standards, processes, and patient outcomes are addressed.

Cultural differences are inevitable, and the best way to manage them and lead our organizations successfully will be to develop **cultural competence**, along with sensitivity. Nurses in today's multicultural society must develop workplaces where diversity flourishes in order to foster a healing environment. Cultural competency will be needed to manage patient care in the future. A good foundation in culturally competent nursing is essential because it may provide a conceptual framework for holistic patient care in a variety of clinical settings and assist the nurse throughout his or her nursing career (Table 3–1).

VALUING DIVERSITY

Nurses often see themselves only in terms of people like themselves. This narrow focus can impede our potential to assist others and pro-

TABLE 3–1

Cultural Norms of the U.S. Health Care System

Beliefs
- Standardized definitions of health and illness
- Omnipotence of technology

Practices
- Maintenance of health and prevention of illness
- Annual physical examinations and diagnostic procedures

Habits
- Charting
- Frequent use of jargon
- Use of a systematic approach and diagnostic procedures

Likes
- Promptness
- Neatness and organization
- Compliance

Dislikes
- Tardiness
- Disorderliness and disorganization

Customs
- Professional deference and adherence to the pecking order found in autocratic and bureaucratic systems
- Use of certain procedures attending birth and death

Rituals
- Physical examination
- Surgical procedures
- Limiting visiting and visitor hours

vide quality health care services. As Figure 3–1 shows, there are many ways in which people differ from one another. The more we know about each other and ourselves, the more likely we are to achieve the goal of helping others grow, develop, and thrive.

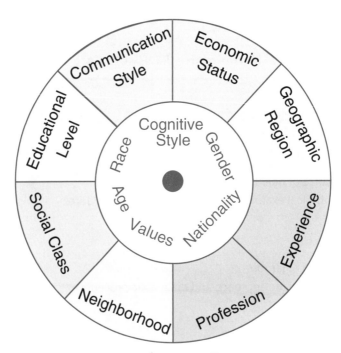

FIGURE 3-1 Ways in which people differ

When nurses consider race, ethnicity, culture, and heritage, they are more sensitive to patients and are therefore able to make better suggestions about patient behavior or wellness. Additionally, when nurses consider the significance of culture, patients are more informed and feel better about their health care provider. As professional health care workers and role models, nurses need to step forward to provide the leadership to ensure that all patients have equal access to quality, culturally appropriate, and culturally competent health care.

What is needed in nursing is a transformation of how culture is understood and the impact it has on health care issues, patient care, and satisfaction levels. This transformation requires nursing leadership to restructure the health care delivery system to support and value differences. New strategies for working with new groups, and evaluating the rewards for valuing those differences will also need to be developed. There is a plan, the Success Model, that may be used in health care to assist in the transformation process discussed earlier. There are four main phases described in the Success Model.

#1 Create a Diversity Vision

Determine where your organization is headed. How will it get there? Is that where you want to go? When will the organization arrive? What does it value? These are the types of questions nurses need to answer before they may focus on a goal. A vision is set and communicated by the leaders in an organization and it trickles down to encompass and encourage staff members.

#2 Build Awareness

Once a vision is in place, the organization may build awareness and commitment. After assessing where the group is, it is possible to take action and focus on building awareness. This phase brings the issue of diversity to all staff members who are most directly affected.

#3 Build Workforce Capability

Awareness is only half the battle. The real benefits from a diverse workforce accrue after organizations learn how to use diversity to their advantage. Focusing on staffing, team building, and communication can do this. Diversity affects each of these areas.

#4 Timely Reinforcement

To keep the organization's awareness operating at a high level, it must be reinforced. Some strategies to reach these ends include formalized norms, established ground rules, and monitoring and measuring success.

Norms and Ground Rules

Every organization has norms, although they are usually unwritten. They reflect the unstated understanding of how things are supposed to happen. They are usually embedded in the organization's character and are accepted by staff members.

Ground rules are more specific than norms. They are generally formally adopted by an organization and describe the way it operates. Successful diverse organizations address diversity through their ground rules, which in turn fosters an environment where staff members of different backgrounds understand one another and work toward the same goals. The following ground rules serve to enhance diversity:

Develop Diversity Awareness

Diversity awareness is a deliberate and conscientious process where the nurse becomes sensitive and appreciative of the values, beliefs, and practices of different cultures and groups.

Expand Cultural Knowledge Base

Cultural knowledge may best be expanded through education regarding other cultures. The goal is to become familiar with culturally and ethnically diverse groups' beliefs, values, and lifestyles.

Develop Cultural Adeptness

Cultural interaction is the process whereby a nurse directly engages with others from culturally diverse backgrounds. Cultural adeptness is the ability to effectively interact with those from different groups. Enhanced cultural skill allows nurses and patients to resolve or head off conflicts when certain culture clashes occur. This effort refines existing knowledge about specific cultural groups, prevents **stereotyping**, and serves as a sound framework for developing a competent cultural style and approach.

Focus on Improvement

There is no need to feel guilty for what has or hasn't been done in the past, even yesterday. Instead, focus on the future. Notice what has happened, figure out how to repair it, and make sure it doesn't happen again.

Self-Awareness

A culturally sensitive nurse is aware of his or her misconceptions. Often, they are one of the main barriers to developing friendships and good working relationships with individuals from other cultures and groups. Unlearning stereotypes is not easy, and it is a lifelong process. It is, however, a very important process.

Nurses must challenge themselves to incorporate selected values, beliefs, lifestyles, and other cultures into their work environment. If nurses believe that every patient is entitled to culturally competent care, then the desire to promote it will be there (Table 3–2).

TABLE 3–2
Strategies for Increasing a Culturally Accepting Environment

- Develop cultural diversity workshops that reflect a cross section of the staff members and patients represented in the organization.
- Include cultural celebrations reflective of the organizational demographics. They can include music, dance, food choices, arts, and traditional dress.
- Make all committees multicultural, especially the ethics committee.
- Include culturally diverse issues on performance evaluations.
- Include cultural diversity sessions in orientation and training programs.
- Provide English as a second language (ESL) classes.
- Provide assertiveness classes for staff members.
- Include legal aspects of defensive charting and health care in the United States in orientation programs.
- Have members do return demonstration on procedures to measure their level of understanding.
- Provide both written and verbal instructions when teaching new organizational policies and procedures.
- Allow extra time for those who need to translate messages into their own language before formulating a reply.
- Speak slowly to non-fluent staff members, and do not use compound or complex sentences. The English language is the only language with contradictions. Avoid using slang or jargon.

Differences and conflicts that occur within a homogenous culture in health care organizations may be intensified for nursing managers in a multicultural workforce. The challenge continues to be the management of a multicultural environment and having staff members view it as an asset (Table 3–3 and Table 3–4).

Cultural competence for nurses must become a habit. Habits are powerful forces and, if used correctly, can be the cohesiveness and order necessary to establish effectiveness in equitable, quality patient care and service provided.

TABLE 3–3

Cultural Diversity Do's

- Develop a cultural habit, the desire to want to effectively build relationships with persons from different cultural backgrounds.
- Recognize that variations exist among all cultural and ethnic groups. This will avoid stereotyping and labeling.
- Become sensitive to nonverbal cues and communications. Be aware that some nonverbal communication may be insulting to specific cultures.
- Remember that ethnicity is only one aspect of cultural diversity. Many factors other than ethnicity constitute a cultural group. Geographical location, gender, age, socioeconomic status, and religion are a few examples.
- Seek out feedback on cross-cultural interactions. Be receptive to constructive criticism and avoid becoming defensive.
- Recognize differences but build on similarities. When members of the group recognize and value differences, they may realize that they are more alike than different.
- Communication is inevitable. Culturally sensitive communication requires knowledge and skill, and awareness of the role one's own culture plays in communicating.
- Cultural competence is a journey, not a destination, but a process of becoming, not being.

TABLE 3–4

Cultural Diversity Don'ts

- Do not assume that because someone looks and behaves the same that there is no cultural difference or barrier to communication.
- Do not rely solely on textbooks, seminars, or printed material for information on cultural groups. Direct interaction will help a person gain accurate information on cultural groups.
- Do not judge others on one's own personal cultures and values. People, as individuals, live by different rules and priorities that are valid to their beliefs.

CULTURALLY SENSITIVE PATIENT CARE

The importance of being culturally sensitive to patients goes beyond language; it is a set of skills that all nurses can learn to use. Some clinical practice settings have felt the impact more heavily than others. Nurses and other health care professionals in every arena can expect to see a continued increase in the number of culturally diverse patient populations (Table 3–5).

The Changing Face of America

Take time to look at the changing face of America and the health care needs of the emerging Hispanic, Asian, Pacific Islander, Indo-Chinese, Vietnamese, and African-American populations. In health care, the educational establishment, the health care delivery system, and consumers are working to provide services that work for the emerging majority.

Providing culturally sensitive care makes sense. Efforts must be made to collaborate with the patient in determining a treatment plan. Unless the health care provider has a sound understanding of the patient's values and perceptions regarding health and illness, their needs cannot be met satisfactorily. The following questions might be a starting point:

- How does the patient view life?
- What are his or her beliefs, values, and norms?
- What is the cultural background and how does it influence behavior?
- How do these factors affect the meaning of health and illness?
- What does health mean in terms of survival?
- How does one person's socialization differ from that of another?

 ASK YOURSELF

Health care professionals continue to speak about the changing face of America. How does the diversity of our society affect access to health care? In what aspects does cultural diversity improve your life? How will medical research be influenced? What about health promotion statistics?

TABLE 3–5

Assessing Your Personal Responses to Transcultural Nursing Situations

When asked to care for a patient from a different cultural background, it is natural to have some concerns. How do you feel about working with patients who are from a very different culture than your own, or who do not speak English? Are you worried that you will not be able to communicate clearly with these patients? Try to respond as honestly as possible to the statements below.

	Agree	Neutral	Disagree
People are the same. I don't behave any differently toward people from a cultural background that differs from mine.	_____	_____	_____
I always know what to say to someone from a different cultural background.	_____	_____	_____
I look forward to caring for a patient from a different cultural background.	_____	_____	_____
I know how to care for a patient who does not speak any English.	_____	_____	_____
I can learn something when I care for patients from diverse cultural backgrounds.	_____	_____	_____
I always introduce myself to the patient's family.	_____	_____	_____
I prefer to care for a patient from my own cultural group who speaks my language because it is easier.	_____	_____	_____

Reprinted with permission of the Association for the Care of Children's Health, 19 Mantua Road, Mt. Royal, NJ 08061, from *Strategies for Working with Culturally Diverse Communities and Clients*, by J. Luckmann.

This understanding and effort promote an awareness of the dimensions and complexities involved in caring for patients from culturally diverse backgrounds. It will also provide a springboard for future considerations as questions and issues arise (Table 3–6).

TABLE 3–6

Cultural Stumbling Blocks

1. Lack of understanding of ethnic groups other than one's own.
2. Stereotyping of members of ethnic groups without consideration of individual differences within the group.
3. Judgment of other ethnic groups according to the standards and values of one's own group.
4. Assignment of negative attributes to the members of other ethnic groups.
5. View of the quality and experiences of other groups as inferior to those of one's own group.

Scope of Care

Cultural factors strongly influence a patient's response to medical intervention and treatment. Cultural beliefs dictate when individuals seek medical care, as well as where they seek it and from whom. Culture also influences patient behaviors in areas of daily life with significant health implications, such as nutrition, medications, hygiene, and self-care.

There is no denying that nurses face challenges when caring for patients from cultural backgrounds different from their own. Some days, just finding a way to bridge the language gap is challenge enough. But it is important to try. Knowing how to work well with patients from different backgrounds makes the best outcome for each patient a real possibility.

Patients develop these values and beliefs to give meaning and predictability to their daily lives. Culturally sensitive health care takes into account the patient's values and beliefs, especially when they conflict with the nurse's personal values and beliefs. Nurses who practice culturally sensitive care are try to focus on the patient's perception of meaningful assistance and the significance of medical and nursing interventions within the context of those values and beliefs.

Care and Values

According to some cultural experts, cultural biases and conflicts may lead to inaccurate diagnosis, inappropriate care and treatment, and misinterpretation of symptoms. There may also be noncompliance and failure to return for follow-up care. Patients may not inform their doctors or nurses of important symptoms, because they are unaware of the need to disclose the information or are not specifically asked.

Additionally, patients may be embarrassed to talk about certain symptoms that are unacceptable in their culture. In some cultures, patients view medical and nursing professionals as authority figures and do not ask questions for fear of appearing disrespectful. A doctor or nurse may give patients instructions without realizing that nodding is a sign of acknowledgment in a particular patient's culture rather than understanding or agreement.

As nurses become more culturally aware of their patient's sensitivities, the areas listed in Table 3–7 may be explored. Exploring these areas during patient assessment provides valuable information about the treatment approach most likely to be accepted and how the treatment plan may best be presented. Patients tend to be more compliant with interventions that comply with their beliefs, and often seek care from doctors and nurses who accept their beliefs about how healing occurs.

Various Approaches to Illness

The standard Western approach to illness, disease, and medical care is a biochemical or structural one, with treatments focusing on correcting abnormal biological or mechanical processes and functions. Many non-Western approaches are very different. They are based on a philosophy of healing that goes beyond the physical. Some individuals, for example, believe that the mind and body are strongly linked. It is noteworthy that the literature of today supports many similar ideas. Other cultures believe that pain and other symptoms are outward manifestations of life events or changes that are meaningful to the patient in a personal, psychological, or religious way.

Many cultures have traditional healing beliefs and methods, known as folk medicine, that have been passed down for generations. These

TABLE 3–7	
Factors That Influence Patient Behavior	
Beliefs about healing	Rituals and practices
Specific cultural values	Beliefs about causes of diseases
Communication preferences	

may include home remedies, rituals, or health practices to prevent unwanted occurrences or to alleviate symptoms. Many of these practices, although not always scientifically proven, have been around for centuries, and some have even been shown to be effective.

Another example may be found in traditional Chinese culture, where collective well-being is most important and individual's needs are often set aside for the benefit of the group. In this case, a patient needing costly medical treatment and resources would forgo treatment if this effort would not benefit the group.

The attitudes of patients and their families toward the ill and disabled also affects their behavior. In traditional Chinese culture, disability and deformity were believed to be punishment from the gods. As a result, disabled family members were kept out of the public, due to shame. Attitudes toward aging and death influence expectations of the elderly, their roles in society, and treatment decisions. In many Asian cultures, elders, considered wise and blessed, hold a special place of honor in the family.

Universal Values

Although there might be differences of opinion regarding diseases, its causes, and treatment, there is a consensus about core values. Table 3–8 outlines these shared values. Although these understandings are shared, cultures often differ in how they prioritize and express them. For example, Hispanics typically make the family the first priority. A patient may decide to attend a family gathering or celebration instead of going to a medical appointment, because not attending the family event would be disrespectful.

Communication

Communication style is another characteristic to consider. Voice quality, volume and speed, facial expression, gesturing, eye contact, body

TABLE 3–8	
Universal Human Values	
Love	Family
Respect	Friendship
Loyalty	Security

distance, and touch, all have different meanings to different people. In traditional Asian cultures, a lowered gaze is often a symbol of respect. Direct eye contact, especially if it is prolonged, is rude. Other cultures are physically expressive, with lots of touch, demonstrative facial expressions, gesturing, and animated speech patterns.

In others, emotions are kept private and not expressed for fear of burdening others or appearing out of control. Stoicism is considered a sign of personal character and strength; patients may not openly acknowledge pain or discomfort. They may even deny the presence of severe pain for fear of appearing weak or lacking in character.

For culturally sensitive care to be given, effective patient communication is critical for accurate diagnosis, the presentation of treatment options, and meaningful patient instruction. Be informed also that it is important to pay attention to a patient's nonverbal clues.

Other Sensitivities

Other areas for nurses to assess include family relationships, perception of the patient being in or out of control, and the patient's orientation to time and place. Some cultures have large networks of extended families, who are all included in meaningful events. In other cultures, the family, not the patient, is given the responsibility for making treatment decisions, especially when the prognosis is serious. Most groups have very clear expectations regarding the behavior and responsibility of family members (Figure 3–2).

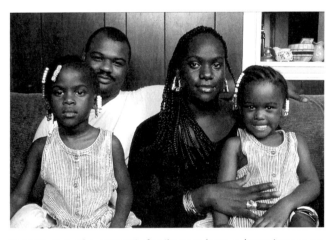

FIGURE 3–2 The patient's family may have a large impact on nursing care.

Implications for Care

It is important to realize that no individual—from any group—lives up to the "textbook" examples of cultural practices and beliefs. Indeed, the various examples provided in this book are not representative of all people of each cultural group mentioned. The level of assimilation, the degree to which individuals take on the characteristics of the dominant society, differs from patient to patient. Factors influencing the rate of assimilation include individual experiences, the strength of family ties, and personal preferences.

There are many variations within groups and many subgroups within groups. As nurses, it is important to remember that each patient is unique and may not fit the expected norm of the group or even belong to the group at all. A patient from a certain cultural background may not practice or subscribe to any of the traditions of that culture. Even patients who appear well assimilated may revert to more traditional cultural behaviors when stressed. Always validate information with patients and continue to evaluate them based on ongoing observations.

PRINCIPLES OF PRACTICE

It is impossible to know the customs of every culture and impractical to study the beliefs of every patient. The following principles, however, may be used to deliver culturally sensitive care to all patients.

Awareness and Sensitivity

Nurses need to exhibit an awareness of and sensitivity to the patient as well as their own values and beliefs. Observing the behaviors of others through one's personal understandings is like looking through a filter or screen. Only by recognizing personal cultural biases is it possible to remove their unintended influence. By being aware that cultures have particular customs and practices, nurses may anticipate problems and suggest alternative options, if needed. Nurses are also well positioned to assess how a treatment may affect a patient's daily life and therefore explore the potential ramifications beforehand (Table 3–9).

Recognition

Nurses experienced with one or two ethnic groups will often recognize certain common customs and behaviors. Patients appreciate this because it eliminates the need for lengthy explanations, minimizes misunderstandings, and creates rapport. Nurses who work with many

TABLE 3–9		

Examining Your Cultural Values

This exercise is designed to help you explore your cultural values (which are most likely Western) in relationship to the cultural values of non-Western cultural groups. This exercise contains nine pairs of statements that have relevance to nursing. The statements on the left represent Western values, whereas the statements on the right represent values held elsewhere in the world. As you rate each statement, *try to be as truthful with yourself as possible.* If you are really honest, you may be surprised at how many of your answers are heavily biased toward Western values.

Directions
Circle 1—If you strongly agree with the statement on the left.
Circle 2—If you agree with the statement on the left.
Circle 3—If you agree with the statement on the right.
Circle 4—If you strongly agree with the statement on the right.

1. Responsible adults prepare for the future and strive to influence events in their lives.	1 2 3 4	Life follows a preordained course. The outcome of events is beyond our control.
2. It is confusing and dishonest to give vague and tentative answers.	1 2 3 4	It is best to avoid direct and honest answers because you may offend and embarrass others.
3. Intelligent, efficient people use their time well and are always punctual.	1 2 3 4	Being punctual to work or a meeting is not as important as enjoying relaxed and pleasant times with family and friends.
4. Stoicism is the appropriate response to severe pain.	1 2 3 4	Loudly crying out and moaning is an appropriate response to severe pain.
5. It is not wise to accept a gift from a person you do not know.	1 2 3 4	It is important to accept gifts and thus avoid insulting the giver.

Table 3–9 *continued*

6. It is a sign of friendliness to address people by their first names.	1 2 3 4	It is disrespectful to address people by their first names unless they give you permission to do so.
7. The best way to gain information is to ask direct questions.	1 2 3 4	It is rude and intrusive to obtain information by asking direct questions.
8. Direct eye contact shows that you are an honest person and that you are interested in the other person.	1 2 3 4	Avoiding direct eye contact may imply that you are not being honest, or you are not interested in what the other person is saying.
9. Ultimately, the needs of the individual are more important than the needs of the family.	1 2 3 4	The needs of the family far outweigh the needs of the individual.

Reprinted with permission of the Association for the Care of Children's Health, 19 Mantua Road, Mt. Royal, NJ 08061, from *Strategies for Working with Culturally Diverse Communities and Clients*, by J. Luckmann.

patients from a particular group may even find it beneficial to study the customs, beliefs, and common health practices of the group. However, guard against the tendency to stereotype members of a certain group, assuming that all group members share beliefs. Just as not all Americans accept the standard Western medical approach to illness and disease, not all members of any other group should be expected to share the common beliefs of that culture.

Respect

By listening to the patient and being open to his or her beliefs, the nurse communicates a respect for the individual and culture. Exploring the use of folk practices and the patient's perception of them will establish rapport and a framework for open communication. The nurse may not understand or agree with a patient's choice of treatment, but accepting the patient's right to choose is the tool that communicates respect. Patients forced to make tough decisions do not need the added burden of harsh judgments or ridicule from others. A climate of cultural sensitivity and respect is instrumental in alleviating patient stress.

Compromise

Acupuncture, biofeedback, and herbal therapies, once considered on the medical fringe, are becoming more accepted today. Considering this, nurses may view these remedies and practices with new insight. If the patient's home remedies are not harmful, they should be explored. If the patient's home remedies are not inherently dangerous and they do not interfere with treatments, simply accept the home remedies as part of the patient's personal healing process. Sometimes, the two may be used together without altering the intended outcome. Nurses often gain the patient's compliance through compromise. After all, even the most established treatment will fail if the patient is uncooperative.

In these times of medical cost containment, the nurse/patient relationship is more important than ever. Culturally sensitive practice has the power to transform nursing care, whether working with patients from other countries or with patients from the United States who have values and beliefs different from our own. Culturally sensitive care enhances the therapeutic relationship, creating a climate in which the patient feels safe and supported to reach optimal wellness.

TRANSCULTURAL ASSESSMENT MODEL

Culturally diverse health care can and should be rendered in a variety of clinical settings. Regardless of the level of care, primary, secondary, or tertiary, a knowledge of the culturally relevant information will assist the nurse in planning and implementing a treatment protocol that is unique for each patient. During the initial assessment, the goal is to summarize the patient data obtained. This information is obtained from a culturally unique individual, the patient. A comprehensive nursing assessment is necessary for both the nurse and the patient to provide culturally appropriate nursing care.

To assist nurses in caring for culturally diverse patients, a transcultural assessment model was developed that focuses on evaluating cultural variables and their impact on health and illness behaviors. In this model, emphasis is placed on the six cultural phenomena evident in all cultural groups as communication, space, social organization, time, environmental control, and biological variations. Each variable is unique and presents a different perspective. As nurses performing assessments, it is important to explore and become knowledgeable about each one in detail.

Communication

Nurses have long realized the importance of communication in the healing process. Communication frequently presents barriers between nurses and their patients, especially when the nurse and patient are from different cultural backgrounds.

A patient who does not understand what is happening or who feels misunderstood may seem angry, noncompliant, or withdrawn. The physical healing process may even be impaired. Nurses may also feel angry and helpless if their communication is not understood or if they cannot understand the patient.

Although communication is universal, nurses should be aware that there are several factors that can influence communication when assessing patients (Table 3–10).

Verbal Communication

Along with vocabulary and grammatical structure, significant communication cues are received from voice quality, tone, rhythm, and speed. Voice quality, which includes pitch and range, can add an important element to communication. The softer volume of Asian-American and Native American speech may be interpreted by the nurse as a shyness.

TABLE 3–10

Factors Influencing Communication

- Physical health and emotional well-being
- Knowledge of the matter or issue being discussed
- Skill at communicating
- Personal needs and interest
- Attitude toward the patient and the subject or issue being discussed
- Background, including cultural, social, and philosophical values
- Personal tendency to make judgments and being judgmental of others
- The environment in which the communication occurs
- Past experiences that relate to the current situation

Tone is an important aspect of the communication message. When patients say they feel fine, they may truly mean that they are in good health; however, it may also mean that they do not feel fine, but they do not wish to discuss it. There is often a latent or hidden meaning in what a person is saying, and the tone frequently provides the clue that is needed to interpret the real message.

Rhythm also varies from culture to culture; some patients have a melodic rhythm to their verbal communication, whereas others appear to lack rhythm. Rhythm may also vary among patients within a culture.

Rate and volume of speech frequently provide a clue to a patient's mood. A depressed patient will tend to talk slowly and quietly, whereas an aggressive, dominating patient is more apt to talk rapidly and loudly.

Patients from some cultural groups may be identified by their dialect, for example, Irish Brogue, or Brooklyn accent. Some African-American dialects include words and expressions not commonly found in standard English.

The meaning of silence also varies among cultural groups. Silences may be thoughtful or they may be blank and empty when the patient has nothing to say. A silence in a conversation can indicate stubbornness and resistance or apprehension and discomfort.

Patients in other cultural groups value silence and view it as essential to understanding their needs. Nurses need to be aware of the possible meaning of silence, so that personal anxiety does not promote the silence being interrupted prematurely or untherapeutically.

Nonverbal Communication

Nonverbal communication also plays an important role in patient relationships. Nonverbal behavior is less significant as isolated behavior, but it does add to the whole message. To fully understand the patient, the nurse may wish to validate impressions with other health team members, because nonverbal behavior is often interpreted differently by people. There may be other behaviors that add to nonverbal behavior and include touch, eye movement, facial expression, and body posture.

Touch, or tactile sensation, has many meanings. It can connect people, provide affirmation, be reassuring, decrease loneliness, share warmth, provide stimulation, and increase self-concept. As a patient, touch is often highly valued and sought after. Nurses need to be aware, however, that touch has cultural significance and symbolism as a learned behavior. Cultural uses of touch vary. In the United States, for example, the mainstream culture generally tolerates hugs and embraces among intimates and a pat on the shoulder as a gesture of camaraderie. In some Native American groups, however, the hand is offered in some interpersonal interactions but the expectation is different; it can be viewed as a gesture of agreement.

Eye movement is used both for observation and to initiate inter-action. The dominant American culture values eye contact as symbolic of a positive self-concept, openness, interest in others, attentiveness, and honesty. Lack of eye movement may therefore be interpreted as a sign of shyness, lack of interest, subordination, humility, guilt, and low self-esteem.

Most African-American and Hispanic patients are comfortable with eye contact and movement. Other groups find eye contact difficult, such as those of the Oriental culture, and some Native Americans who relate eye contact and movement to an invasion of privacy and to impoliteness.

Facial expression also varies with culture. Italian, Jewish American, African-American, and Hispanic patients smile readily and use many facial expressions, along with gestures and words, to communicate feelings of happiness, pain, and displeasure. Facial expression can also be used to convey an opposite meaning of one that is felt; some patients of the Oriental culture display negative emotions concealed with a smile.

Communication is also affected by body posture. It can provide important messages about receptivity. Matching body movements to those of another person can communicate a sense of solidarity, even if solidarity is not present. Rigid muscles, flexed body, and cautious movements communicate physical pain. Knowledge of sociocultural heritage is essential in interpreting body language, because various body parts are used differently in different cultures.

Space

A patient's comfort level is related to personal space, and discomfort is experienced when space is invaded. Although personal space is an individual matter and varies with the situation, dimensions of the per-sonal space comfort zone also vary from culture to culture. It is impor-tant for nurses to remember that territoriality, or the need for space, serves four functions: security, privacy, autonomy, and self-identity.

Security includes actual safety from harm and gives the patient a feeling of being safe. The nurse should remember that if a patient is in a safe place where there is a feeling of control, he or she will feel less threatened, and less anxious. A patient who is hospitalized is out of his or her comfortable surroundings and lacks control. The patient often perceives that his or her automony is threatened when asked personal questions that require sharing of feelings and thoughts.

Social Organization

Cultural behavior, or how a patient acts in certain situations, is socially acquired and not generically inherited. Patterns of cultural behavior are important to the nurse because they provide explanations for behaviors.

When nurses provide care to patients from a sociocultural background other than their own, they should have an awareness of and sensitivity to the patient's sociocultural background, including knowledge of family structure, religious values and beliefs, and how ethnicity and culture relate to role assignment within the group.

Any social organization or group may be viewed as the environment where the patient strives for health. This environment not surprisingly often contains extended families. It is important for the nurse to recognize that other family members may also need intervention.

Whether the family is viewed as an environment or as a patient, the nurse needs to incorporate cultural concepts when developing the nursing plan of care. The nursing process is used regardless of how the patient is viewed. The differences that occur are the result of cultural variables and beliefs that are common to particular ethnic groups. The nurse must recognize these differences.

Time

The concept of time is very familiar to most individuals regardless of cultural heritage. Appreciating cultural differences about time is important for the nurse. When patients of different cultures interact in the health care setting, there is a great potential for misunderstanding. If nurses are to avoid misreading issues that involve time perceptions, they must have an understanding of how other individuals in different cultures view time (Table 3–11).

The nurse who understands time as a cultural variable with a significant impact on patients will also gain an understanding of how time is managed to give quality patient care.

TABLE 3–11	
Time and Ethnicity	
American	Future over present
Southern Black	Present over future
Puerto Rican	Present over future
Southern Appalachian	Present
Mexican American	Present
Traditional Chinese American	Present

Environmental Control

Environmental control can refer to the patient's perception of his ability to direct factors in the environment. In the broadest sense, health care may be viewed as a balance between the individual and the environment. Health practices such as eating nutritiously and subscribing to preventive health services available in the community are believed to have a positive effect on the individual.

Some cultures believe in a direct connection between the body and the forces of nature; therefore, it is important for the nurse to recognize the relevance of natural phenomena such as phases of the moon, positions of the planets, and seasons of the year. Some people from other cultural groups use the zodiac signs to manipulate health protocols but do not mention this to health professionals for fear of being ridiculed.

The presence of an alternative medical or folk medicine system that is different from, and possibly in direct conflict with, the Western medical system can serve to complicate matters. It not only becomes a matter of offering health care in the place of no health care, or offering superior care in lieu of inferior care, but the nurse must remember that some persons from diverse settings have deeply ingrained beliefs about how to attain and maintain health.

These beliefs, which may be linked to the natural and supernatural worlds, may adversely affect the physician and patient and nurse and patient relationships and thus influence the patient's decision to follow or not to follow prescribed treatment plans and protocols. It is important for the nurse to determine what the patient has already tried regarding home remedies and what he or she has been doing to combat the illness.

Biological Variations

Culture is often used to describe a person's beliefs and norms. Race, by contrast, is held to describe one's genetic or biological makeup—skin color, hair, eye color, and other features. When working with patients from diverse cultural backgrounds, the nurse must also be aware of racial implications (Table 3–12).

Skin color is an important feature and is often an important biological variation in terms of nursing care. As nursing care delivery is based on accurate patient assessment, a darker skin color may be more difficult to assess if there are color changes. When nurses care for patients with highly pigmented skin, the nurse must first establish the baseline skin color.

TABLE 3–12

Major Differences in Diseases and Various Groups' Susceptibility

- African Americans, Native American Indians, Asian and Pacific Islanders account for nearly two thirds of the cases of tuberculosis reported.
- Diabetes is a major health problem across races and genders, except in Alaskan Eskimos. The prevalence increases with age and at all ages is highest among African-American women.
- Incidence of hypertension is reported higher in African Americans; it is more severe and associated with a higher mortality rate in African Americans.
- Sickle cell anemia is the most common genetic disorder in the United States, which occurs predominantly in African Americans.
- Systemic lupus erythematosus affects women more often than men; and it occurs more frequently among African Americans. It is extremely rare among the Asian population.
- AIDS is higher among Hispanics and African Americans, although cases are increasing in all populations.

The best time for this activity is during daylight hours. Dark-skinned patients should be given a bed near light for better visual assessment. If daylight is not available, a lamp with at least a 60-watt bulb should be used.

To establish a baseline skin color, the nurse must observe those skin surfaces that have the least amount of pigmentation, which include the surfaces of the forearms, the palms of the hands, the soles of the feet, the abdomen, and the buttocks. When observing these areas the nurse should look for an underlying red tone, which is present in all skin, regardless of color. Absence of this red tone may indicate pallor.

Additional areas that are important to assess in dark-skinned patients may include the mouth, the conjunctiva, and the nail beds. Generally speaking, the darkness of the oral mucosa correlates with the patient's skin color. The darker the skin, the darker the mucosa; nevertheless, the mucosa is lighter than the skin. The conjunctiva reflect the color changes of cyanosis or pallor. It is also a good site for observing petechiae.

Nail beds are an important area to assess and are useful in attempting to detect cyanosis or pallor. In dark-skinned patients, it may be difficult to assess the nail beds because they may be highly pigmented, thick, lined, or contain melanin deposits. Regardless of color, it is important for the nurse to note how quickly the color returns to the nail beds after pressure has been released from the free edge of the nail.

In terms of genetic variations, the basic genetic makeup of a patient is determined from the moment of conception and is considered that person's race. Although race may be irrelevant in some situations, knowing the racial predisposition to a certain disease is often helpful in evaluating patients and diagnosing their illnesses and assessing risk factors. The increased or decreased incidence of a particular disease may be genetically determined.

The concept of cultural competence in nursing is exciting. It is beginning to expand as nurses incorporate culturally appropriate care in daily nursing assignments. Understanding diversity, and the ability to complement one another, allows nurses to accept and appreciate the impact of culture on health care. Table 3–13 provides a useful guide for many cultural characteristics and values. Bear in mind, however, that only general information is provided and there are variations within any group.

TABLE 3–13   Cultural Characteristics and Health Care Beliefs and Practices

Cultural Group	Communication Styles	Family, Social, and Work Relationships	Health Values and Beliefs	Health Customs and Practices
Asian-American Chinese	Nonverbal and contextual cues important. Silence after a statement is used by a speaker who wishes the listener to consider the importance of what is said. Self-expression repressed. Value silence. Touching limited. May smile when do not understand. Hesitant to ask questions.	Hierarchical, extended family pattern. Deference to authority figures and elders. Both parents make decisions about children. Value self-reliance and self-restraint. Important to preserve family's honor and save face. Value working hard and giving to society.	Health viewed as gift from parents and ancestors and the result of a balance between the energy forces of yin (cold) and yang (hot). Illness caused by an imbalance. Blood is the source of life and cannot be regenerated. Lack of blood and chi (innate energy) produces debilitation and long illness. Respect for the body and belief in reincarnation dictates that one must die with the body intact. Believe a good physician can accurately diagnose an illness by simply examining a person using the senses of sight, smell, touch, and listening.	May use medical care system in conjunction with Chinese methods of acupuncture (a yin treatment consisting of the insertion of needles to meridians to cure disease or relieve pain) and moxibustion (a yang treatment during which heated, pulverized wormwood is applied to appropriate meridians to assist with labor and delivery and other yin disorders). Medicinal herbs, e.g., ginseng, are widely used. Fear painful, intrusive diagnostic tests, especially the drawing of blood. May refuse intrusive surgery or autopsy. May be distrustful of physicians who order and use painful or intrusive diagnostic tests. Accept immunizations as valid means of disease prevention. Heavy use of condiments such as mono-sodium glutamate and soy sauce.

Cultural Group	Communication Styles	Family, Social, and Work Relationships	Health Values and Beliefs	Health Customs and Practices
Japanese	Attitude, action, and feeling more important than words. Tend to listen empathically. Touching limited. Direct eye contact considered a lack of respect. Stoic; suppress overt emotion. Value self-control, politeness, and personal restraint.	Close, interdependent, intergenerational relationships. Individual needs subordinate to family's needs. Will endure great hardship to ensure success of next generation. Belonging to right clique or society important to status and success. Obligation to kin and work group. Education highly valued.	Believe illness caused by contact with polluting agents (e.g., blood, skin diseases, corpses), social or family disharmony, or imbalance from poor health habits. Cleanliness highly valued.	Tend to rely on Euro-American medical system for preventive and illness care. Oldest adult child responsible for care of elderly. Care of disabled is a family's responsibility. Take pride in good health of children. Believe in removal of diseased areas. Practice of emotional control may make pain assessment more difficult. When visiting ill, often bring fruit or special Japanese foods.
Vietnamese	Respect and harmony most important values. Disrespectful to question authority figures. Avoid direct eye contact. Strong focus on respect through use of titles and terms indicating family and generational relationships. Modesty of speech and action valued.	Family close, multigenerational, and primary social network. Filial piety of primary importance. Father is family decision maker. Individual needs are subordinate to family's needs. Training of children shared by extended family. Behavior of individual reflects on total family. Education highly valued.	Believe illness caused by naturalistic (bad food, water), supernaturalistic (punishment for displeasing a deity), metaphysical (imbalance of hot and cold) forces, or from contamination by germs.	Often use both folk and some parts of the scientific health care system such as drugs. Family orally transmits folk medicine information. Health care regarded as family responsibility. Use medicinal herbs, therapeutic diets, hygienic measures to promote health, prevent illness, and treat illness. All means and resources available to family are tried before seeking outside help.

continues

Table 3–13 *continued*

Cultural Group	Communication Styles	Family, Social, and Work Relationships	Health Values and Beliefs	Health Customs and Practices
Vietnamese *continued*	Relaxed concept of time; punctuality less significant than propriety. Use Ya to indicate listening, not understanding. Avoid asking direct questions.			Folk care practices include *cao gio* (rubbing skin with coin) for respiratory illnesses, *bat gil* (skin pinching) for headaches, inhalation of aromatic oils and liniments for respiratory and gastrointestinal illnesses. May consult priest, astrologer, shaman, or fortune-teller for prediction or instruction about health, or use hot and cold foods and substances to restore balance.
Filipinos	Personal dignity and preserving self-esteem highly valued. Nonverbal communication important. Eye contact avoided. Avoid direct expressions of disagreement, particularly with authority figures. Sex, socioeconomic status, and tuberculosis too personal to discuss. Need to engage in "small talk" before discussing more serious matters.	Multigenerational matrifocal family with strong family ties. Avoid behavior that shames family. Defer to elderly. Individual interests subordinate to family's interests. Value interpersonal relationships over current events.	Tend to believe illness is related to natural (unhealthy environment), supernatural (God's will and providence), and metaphysical (imbalance between hot and cold) forces. Tend to be fatalistic in outlook on life.	If accessible, may use both folk and scientific medical systems. Folk practices include flushing (stimulating perspiration, vomiting, bowel evacuation), heating (hot and cold substances to maintain internal body temperature), and protection (use of amulets, good luck pieces, religious medals, pictures, statues). Tend to be stoic; believe pain is God's will and He will give one the strength to bear it.

Cultural Group	Communication Styles	Family, Social, and Work Relationships	Health Values and Beliefs	Health Customs and Practices
Black Americans				
African Americans	Many have high level of caution or distrust of majority group. Expressive use of nonverbal behavior and speech. Many use an English dialect: "black English." Very sensitive to lack of congruence between verbal and nonverbal messages. Value direct eye contact. May "test" health professionals before submitting self to decisions and care of the majority group's health care providers.	Strong kinship bonds in extended family. 50% patriarchical; 50% matriarchical families. Large social networks of family and unrelated members. Elderly members respected, particularly maternal grandparents. Strong sense of peoplehood; come to aid of others in crisis. Black minister a strong influence in community. Women protect health of family. Worth of education is judged by its "usability in living."	Illness is a collective event that disrupts the total family system. Illness believed to be a natural event resulting from conflict or disharmony in one's life, failure to protect oneself from cold air, pollution, food, and water, or sent by God as punishment. Those more assimilated to dominant culture perceive illness to be due to preventable injury or pathology.	Health is maintained by proper diet, rest, clean environment. Self-care and folk medicine (usually religious in origin) very prevalent. Individuals from more rural backgrounds are more likely to use folk practitioners. Attempt home remedies first; may not seek help from the medical establishment until illness serious; often will elect to retain dignity rather than seek care if values and sensibilities are demeaned. Prayer is common means for prevention and treatment. When ill or hospitalized, visits by family minister are sought, expected, and valued to help cope with illness and suffering.
Haitians	New immigrants and older persons often speak only Haitian Creole. Hand gesturing and tone of voice frequently used to complement speech. Smiling and nodding often do not indicate understanding.	Two-class social system: wealthy and poor. Rural and poor families tend to be matriarchical. Children taught unquestioning obedience to adults. Child-rearing shared by parents and older siblings.	Illness believed to be caused by supernatural forces (angry spirits, enemies, or the dead) or natural forces (irregularities of blood volume, flow, viscosity, purity, color or temperature [hot and cold]; gas [gaz]; movement and consistency of mother's milk; hot/cold	Use medical care and folk medicine simultaneously. Health maintained by good dietary and hygienic habits. Adherence to prescribed treatments directly related to perceived severity of illness; resist dietary and activity restrictions.

continues

Table 3-13 *continued*

Cultural Group	Communication Styles	Family, Social, and Work Relationships	Health Values and Beliefs	Health Customs and Practices
Haitians *continued*	Direct eye contact used in formal and casual conversations. Unassertive — will not ask questions if health care provider appears busy or rushed. Touch is perceived as comforting, sympathetic, and reassuring.	Tend to be status conscious, thus parents often choose children's mate to increase family status.	imbalance in the body; bone displacement). Believe health is a personal responsibility.	Hot and cold and light and heavy properties of food are used to gain harmony with one's life cycle and bodily states. Natural illnesses are first treated by home remedies. Supernatural illnesses treated by healers: herbalist or leaf doctor (*dokte fey*), midwife (*fam saj*), or voodoo priest (*houngan*), or priestess (*mambo*). Use amulets and prayer to protect against supernatural illnesses.
Hispanic Americans Mexicans	Most bilingual; may use non-standard English. Introductory embrace common. Tend to revert to native language in times of stress. Consider prolonged eye contact disrespectful but value direct eye contact.	Strong kinship bonds among nuclear and extended families including *compadres* (godparents). Strong need for family group togetherness. Respect wisdom of elders. Children highly desired and valued; accompany family everywhere.	Illness can be prevented by: being good, eating proper foods, and working proper amount of time; also accomplished through prayer, wearing religious medals or amulets, and sleeping with relics at home.	Magico-religious practices common. Usually seek help from older women in family before going to a Jerbero, who specializes in the use of herbs and spices to restore balance/health or *curandero* or *curandera* (holistic healers) with whom they have a uniquely personal relationship and share a common worldview. Prevent and treat illness with "hot" and "cold" food prescriptions and prohibitions.

Cultural Group	Communication Styles	Family, Social, and Work Relationships	Health Values and Beliefs	Health Customs and Practices
Mexicans *continued*	Appreciate "small talk" before initiating actual conversation topic. Appreciate a nondirective approach with open-ended questions. Hesitant to talk about sex but may do so more freely with nurse of same sex. Father should be present when speaking with a male child.	Entire family contributes to family's financial welfare. Homes frequently decorated with statues, medals, and pictures of saints. Children often reluctant to share communal showers in schools. Relaxed concept of time.	Some believe illness is due to: body imbalance between *caliente* (hot) and *frío* (cold) or "wet" and "dry"; dislocation of parts of the body (*empacho* — ball of food stuck to the stomach wall or *caída de la mollera* — more serious, depression of fontanelle in infant); magic or supernatural (*mal ojo* [evil eye] or punishment from God); strong emotional state (*susto* — soul loss following an extreme fright); or *envidia* (success leads to envy by others resulting in misfortune). More concerned with present than with future and therefore may focus on immediate solutions rather than long-term goals. May view hospital as place to go to die.	For severe illness, use scientific medical system but also make promises, visit shrines, use medals and candles, offer prayers — elements of Catholic and Pentecostal rituals and artifacts. Extreme modesty; may avoid seeking medical care and open discussions of sex. Children and adults expected to and do endure pain stoically.
Puerto Ricans	Older, newly moved to the mainland often speak only Spanish; others usually bilingual.	Paternalistic, hierarchical family; father is family provider and decision maker. Family of central importance.	Many believe illness is caused by imbalance of hot and cold, evil spirits, and forces.	Use folk practitioners and medical establishment or both.

continues

Table 3-13 *continued*

Cultural Group	Communication Styles	Family, Social, and Work Relationships	Health Values and Beliefs	Health Customs and Practices
Puerto Ricans *continued*	May use nonstandard English. Personal and family privacy valued. Consider questions regarding family disrespectful and presumptuous. Tend to have a relaxed sense of time.	Families usually large. Parents demand absolute obedience and respect from children. Women in family tend to all ill members and dispense all medicines. Children valued — seen as gift from God.	Many believe in spirits and spiritualism, having visions, and hearing voices. Accept many idiosyncratic behaviors; often perceive behavioral disturbances as symptoms of illness that need to be treated rather than judged. Suspicious and fearful of hospitals.	When ill: first seek advice from women in family; if not sufficient, seek help from a *señora* (woman especially knowledgeable about causes and treatment of common illnesses); if unable to help, consult an *espiritista, curandera,* or *santeria* (if psychiatric problem) who listens nonjudgmentally; often use herbs, lotions, salves, and massage and *caliente* (hot), *fresco* (cool), and *frio* (cold) treatments; if no relief, may go to a medical physician; if not satisfied, may return to any of the preceding.
Cuban Americans	Most new immigrants are bilingual. Expect some social talk before getting to actual reason for discussion.	Strong family and maternal and paternal kinship ties. Mother tends to explain and reason constantly to obtain child's conformity to family norms. Elderly cared for at home. Mother primary health care provider in home and must be included in all health education programs for family members.	Believe good health results from prevention and good nutrition. Believe plump babies and young children are most healthy and admirable.	Combine use of medical practitioners with religious and nonreligious folk practitioners. Tend to be eclectic in health-seeking practices and, in some instances, may seek assistance of *santeros* (Afro-Cuban healers) and *espiritista* to complement treatment by medical practitioners. Parents very concerned about eating habits of their children; may spend a considerable part of the family budget on food.

Cultural Group	Communication Styles	Family, Social, and Work Relationships	Health Values and Beliefs	Health Customs and Practices
Cuban Americans *continued*		Children often supported and assisted by parents long after becoming adults. Extensive network of support for family and family members from social institutions such as schools, health clinics, and social clubs. Ambitious and take advantage of any opportunity to be successful in their work.		
American Indians	Most speak their Indian language and English. Nonverbal communication important. Unwavering eye gaze viewed as insulting. Tend to take time to form an opinion of health professionals. Consider silence essential to understanding and respecting another. A pause following a question signifies that the question is important enough to be given thoughtful consideration.	Strong extended family and kinship structure — usually including relatives from both sides of the family. Believe family members are responsible for one another. Elder members greatly respected and assume leadership roles. Children valued. Children taught respect for traditions and to honor wisdom and those who possess it.	Medicine and religion strongly interwoven. Believe health results from being in harmony with nature and universe. Reject germ theory as cause of illness; believe every sickness and pain is a price to be paid for something that occurred in the past or will happen in the future. May carry objects believed to guard against witchcraft.	Use total immersion in water, sweat lodges, and special rituals in the gathering, preparation, and use of herbs to regain harmony and thus health. Diviner-diagnosticians determine cause of illness, recommend treatment, and refer to a specific medicine man — diagnose but do not have powers or skill to implement medical treatment. Medicine man — traditional healer in whom most faith placed — uses herbs and special chants and rituals to cure illness. Singers effect cures by laying on of hands and by the power of the songs they obtain from supernatural beings.

continues

Table 3–13 *continued*

Cultural Group	Communication Styles	Family, Social, and Work Relationships	Health Values and Beliefs	Health Customs and Practices
American Indians *continued*	Hesitant to discuss personal affairs until trust is developed, which can take some time. Believe it is ethically wrong to speak for another person. Hesitant to talk about sex but may do so more freely with a nurse of the same sex. Sensitive about having their words and behavior written down.			
Middle Eastern	Men and women do not shake hands or touch each other in any manner outside immediate family or marital relationship. Touching and embracing on arrival and on departure are common among same sex. Use silence to show respect for another.	Providing family care and support is an important responsibility. Male-dominated. Eldest male is the decision maker. Male children valued more than females. Adult male must not be alone with any female except wife.	Magico-religious; follow will of Allah — passive role is norm. Various beliefs about the causes of disease coexist: "hot" and "cold" and "evil eye." Physically robust person considered healthier. Emotional distress expressed as "heart disease." Obligation and responsibility to visit the sick, help others when they are ill, especially children and elderly.	Use magico-religious, folk, self-care, and medical science. Use amulets inscribed with verses of the Koran, turquoise stones, charm of a hand with five fingers to enhance protective powers against evil eye. Male health professionals prohibited from touching or examining a female patient. May refuse to have female health professionals care for males. The dead must be buried with the body intact.

Cultural Group	Communication Styles	Family, Social, and Work Relationships	Health Values and Beliefs	Health Customs and Practices
Middle Eastern *continued*			Expect immediate pain relief from health professionals.	May perform female circumcision to ensure Muslim females become "good wives" and are accepted by other women in the family and community.
White Americans Euro-Americans (middle class)	Often separate into male and female groups at social events unless the activity is for couples. Nod to denote understanding or indicate agreement. Tend to maintain a "neutral" facial expression in public. Tolerate hugs and embraces among intimates and close friends. Pat on shoulder denotes camaraderie; firm handshake symbolic of goodwill. Good social manners include smiling, speaking pleasantly and warmly to put the other person at ease. Insist on own personal space.	Nuclear family professed norm. Two primary family goals: encourage and nurture each individual, produce healthy, autonomous children. Power more egalitarian. Socialize primarily with work-related and neighborhood friends. Generosity in time of crisis. Espouse the Protestant work ethic: work and plan for the future. Competitive and achievement oriented. Value education and knowledge from books as well as from experience.	Generally future oriented and believe one's internal and external environments can be controlled. Expect the most modern medical technology to be used when ill. Believe good health is a personal responsibility. Accept the germ theory and perceive illness to be the result of injury or pathology that can usually be prevented or contained through individual lifestyle and community health efforts.	Engage in self-care practices: strive for balanced diet, rest and activity, and work and leisure. Utilize self-care over-the-counter remedies for minor illnesses. Utilize medical health care system and health professionals for health screening, illness care, and follow-up. Intolerant of delays in health care services and of health professionals whose practices they believe are out of date. Read and access other media sources to increase understanding of risk factors, health promotion practices, and treatment techniques. Want to be consulted by health professionals before treatment is initiated but tend to accept health professionals' medical and health care judgments.

continues

Table 3–13 *continued*

Cultural Group	Communication Styles	Family, Social, and Work Relationships	Health Values and Beliefs	Health Customs and Practices
Appalachian	Avoid answering questions related to income, children's school attendance, the affairs of others in the household and of neighbors. May consider direct eye contact impolite or aggressive. Uncomfortable with the impersonal and bureaucratic orientation of the American health system. May evaluate health professional on basis of interpersonal skills rather than on professional competence.	Community interdependence. Stay near home for protection. Keep ties with kin. Guard against strangers and outsiders. Kindness to others valued. Do more for others, less for self.	Disability an inevitable part of life and aging. Severity of illness perceived in terms of degree of dependency it necessitates during the period of illness. Believe cold and lack of personal care cause illness. Frugal; always use home remedies first. The hospital is "the place where people die."	Use folk practices "first and last." Rule for primary prevention: "eat right, take fluids, keep the body strong, stay warm when it's cold." Self-care for minor illnesses. Medical care for serious illnesses. Help from kin as needed for primary care. Help from family members and extended family expected and accepted.

Compiled from information in Giger, J. N., & Davidhizar, R. E. (1995). *Transcultural nursing: Assessment and intervention* (2nd ed.). Baltimore: Mosby; Leininger, M. M. (1994). *Transcultural nursing: Concepts, theory, research, and practice* (2nd ed.). Columbus, OH: McGraw Hill and Greyden Press; Geissler, E. (1994). *A pocket guide to cultural assessment.* Baltimore: Mosby; Spector, R. E. (1991). *Cultural diversity in health and illness* (3rd ed.). Norwalk, CT: Appleton & Lange; and Wong, D. L. (1995). *Whaley and Wong's nursing care of infants and children* (5th ed.). Baltimore: Mosby.

KEY POINTS

- Culture is the set of values, beliefs, and traditions held by a specific group that is learned and handed down from generation to generation.
- One's culture guides behavior, is primarily transmitted through language, and can be adapted over time.
- Ethnic groups are made up of people who share common and unique cultural and social beliefs and social patterns.
- As members of a minority live within a dominant group, cultural characteristics often are lost through assimilation.
- A wide variety of cultural and ethnic characteristics affect transcultural nursing care. These characteristics include family member roles, communication, nutrition, and income levels.
- Certain physiological and psychological characteristics that are found in specific cultural and ethnic groups are risk factors for illness.
- The health care system is a culture, with nursing being the largest subculture.
- As part of the health care system, which has its own values and behaviors, nurses must be aware of the tendency of health care professionals toward cultural imposition and ethnocentrism.
- Guidelines for transcultural nursing care help the nurse accept the values, beliefs, and behaviors of others.
- When nurses provide transcultural care, they demonstrate cultural sensitivity by recognizing and respecting cultural diversity.

CRITICAL THINKING ACTIVITIES

1. In the acute care hospital setting, you are caring for a patient who has a cultural background different from your own. Explain how you would assess the patient's beliefs and practices in developing the individualized care plan. Discuss the importance of exploring your personal feelings about the differences in cultural backgrounds.

2. Rosa Salazar is a refugee from El Salvador who now lives in California and has residency status in the United States. Several weeks ago she underwent a mastectomy. Señora Calderon has recently experienced menopause. She lives with her husband in a small suburb of Los Angeles, fairly near her two grown sons and their families. Critically analyze the cultural factors that are

important to consider in providing care to Señora Calderon. For example, how does Latin American culture view breast surgery? Menopause? How might you assist her in meeting her developmental tasks? What will be some problems that Señora Salazar might encounter in the U.S. health care system?

➠ CASE STUDY

Maria Gonzalez, a new graduate nurse argues with her supervisor, certain that her rational approach will win her case. Family members of one of Maria's patients have become a familiar nursing "problem" for the staff on the nursing unit. Arriving in "unreasonably large groups," several adults, adolescent family members, and younger children often come to visit Mrs. Garcia, mother and grandmother. The problem of overnight accommodation for the family has become a topic of lively debate among the nursing staff. Sensitive to the cultural practices of the patient and family, the new graduate begins her argument on behalf of the family's right to adhere to their cultural practices. The supervisor listens as Maria argues her case for cultural sensitivity.

The nature of the nursing problem is complex and multifaceted. Discuss the interconnectedness of the various components of the situation. Consider the values and beliefs of both the nurses within the health care delivery system and the family's extended social network. What suggestions might the supervisor give to Maria? Discuss possible referral resources that may be able to provide some assistance.

BIBLIOGRAPHY

Andrews, M. M., & Boyle, J. S. (Eds.). (1995). *Transcultural concepts in nursing care* (2nd ed). Philadelphia: Lippincott-Raven.

Bakker, L. (1995). *Communicating across cultures.* Albany, New York: Crest Books.

Davidhizer, R., & Giger, J. (1995). *Transcultural nursing: Assessment and intervention.* St. Louis: Mosby Publishing.

Dienemann, J. (Ed.). (1997). *Cultural diversity in nursing issues, strategies, outcomes.* Waldorf, MD: American Nurses Publishing.

Leininger, M. (Ed.). (1995). *Transcultural nursing: Concepts, theories, research and practices* (2nd ed.). Columbus, OH: McGraw Hill.

Lenburg, C. B. (Ed.). (1998). *Promoting cultural competence in and through nursing education: A critical review and comprehensive plan for action.* Philadelphia, PA: Lippincott-Rauen.

Meleis, A. I. (Ed.). (1998). *Diversity, marginalization, and culturally competent health care: Issues in knowledge development.*

Purnell, L. D. (Ed.). (1998). *Transcultural health care: A culturally based approach.* Philadelphia: F. A. Davis Company.

Spector, R. (Ed.). (1996). *Cultural diversity in health and illness, guide to heritage assessments and health traditions.* Stanford, CT: Appleton & Lange.

Tripp-Reimer, T. (1995). *Cultural assessment: A multidimensional approach.* Monterey, CA: Wadsworth Publishing.

INTERNET RESOURCES

Cultural Competency: A Journey
  http://www.bphc.hrsa.dhhs.gov/culturalcompetence
EthnoMed homepage
  http://www.healthlinks.washington.edu/clinical/ethnomed
Georgetown University Child Development Center—National Center for Cultural Competence
  http://www.dml.georgetown.edu/depts/pediatrics/
Transcultural Nursing Diversity in Health and Illness
  http://www.megalink.net/~vic/
Transcultural Nursing Society
  http://www.tcns.org

CHAPTER **4**

Nursing and the Law

OVERVIEW

Health care professionals delivering services to health care consumers must practice within the limits of federal and state legislation. These laws, or standards, should govern every nurse's behavior. This chapter discusses the sources of the law, standards of care, and nurse practice and licensure. Definitions of health care rendered by the courts and precedent setting decisions affect how, when, where, and to whom health care will be provided. The legal process, malpractice insurance, and documentation issues will be discussed.

OBJECTIVES

Upon completion of this chapter, the reader should be able to:

- Describe the components of the legal process.
- Discuss the sources of the law.
- Describe general legal issues affecting nursing practice.
- Explore the legal relationship between the patient and the nurse.
- Describe standards of care.
- Discuss the terms *negligence* and *malpractice*.
- Discuss the four elements of malpractice.

⇒ **KEY TERMS**

Breach of duty	Malpractice
Crime	Negligence
Duty	Standards of care
Informed consent	Tort

INTRODUCTION

As changes in our society occur, standards of morality and ethics become fluid. At any given moment, different views about morality or ethics may not conform to the letter of the law. This is particularly true in health care and other areas of society where technology has had a major impact. In these areas technology is moving much faster than our moral and legal standards can evolve. As a result, the law may be unclear. It may not provide specific answers to a difficult health care dilemma. Nevertheless, nurses have a responsibility to understand the current legal and ethical guidelines that govern patient care.

A nurse who understands the legal process may look at societal issues and respond to problems with confidence. The laws provide fundamental rights and establish relationships between the nurse and the patient. The validity of the legislation passed and the regulations established is measured against federal or state constitutional standards, or both, depending on the issue in question.

SOURCES OF THE LAW

There are four main sources of laws or rules of conduct in the United States. These sources are the constitution, the legislatures, the judiciary, and administrative regulations.

Constitution

In the United States, the constitution of the federal government and that of each state indicate how their government is credited and given authority. These documents state the principles and provisions for establishment of specific laws. Although they themselves contain relatively few laws (called constitutional law), they are constant guides to legislative bodies. On the local level, each state constitution directs the governing of a specific geographic area, but it cannot violate the principles set down in the federal constitution.

Although individuals cede certain rights in order that a government may be created, the constitutions are not without their limits. For example, the first ten amendments of the federal constitution are referred to as the Bill of Rights. These amendments restrict the passage of laws that infringe on certain basic liberties. These include freedom of worship, freedom of speech, and freedom from unwarranted search and seizure of our homes and persons. Each state constitution sets similar limitations.

The Legislatures

The various constitutions of the United States created legislative bodies that are responsible for enacting laws. A law enacted by a legislative body is commonly held to be part of either statutory or public law. These laws must be in keeping with the federal constitution as well. The Nurse Practice Acts are statutory laws.

The Judiciary

Most governments also provide for a judiciary system responsible for reconciling controversies and conflicts. It interprets legislation as it has been applied in specific instances and makes decisions in relation to law enforcement. Over the years, a body of law known as common law, private law, or civil law, has grown out of these accumulated judiciary decisions.

Common law is based on the principle known as *stare decisis* or "let the decision stand." In other words, once a decision has been made in a court of law, that decision becomes the rule to follow when other cases involving similar circumstances and facts arise. The case that first sets down the rule by decision is called a precedent. Court decisions may be changed but only when strong justification exists. Common law helps prevent one set of rules being used to judge one person, and another set being used to judge another person in similar circumstances.

Common law is directly concerned with nursing. For example, operating under common law, student nurses in hospital-controlled schools of nursing are considered employees of the hospital.

Administrative Regulations

Outside of the judiciary or legislative arena, a nurse's actions are governed by administrative rules and regulations. These are enforceable

ASK YOURSELF

As a student nurse, when the hospital's or any clinical site's policy conflicts with the nurse practice act, what should you do? If as a nursing student you violate the state board's practice act, what are the implications for your future nursing career?

just as any law in the country. They are referred to as administrative law.

Examples of federal administrative agencies include the Federal Trade Commission, the Federal Communications Commission, and Interstate Commerce Commission. The boards of nursing are examples of administrative agencies at the state level.

STANDARDS OF CARE

Standards of care are those acts that are permitted or prohibited to be performed by a prudent person working within the parameters of his or her education, license, experience, and the conditions existing at the time. Standards of care are determined or established by professional organizations, the nurse practice acts of each state, guidelines established by accrediting bodies or hospitals, nursing homes, educational programs, and health care professionals.

One of the functions of the law applied to nursing practice is to define the standard of care that nurses must provide. All states have nurse practice acts that define the scope of nursing practice in their particular state.

Standards of care maintain that it is the nurse's duty to a patient to provide reasonable, prudent care required by the circumstances. These standards are the ruler against which a nurse's performance is measured. Standards of care concern nurses' accountability or obligations to account for their actions. All nurses should know the standards of care they are expected to meet.

Institutions or agencies have their own policies and procedures that define the agency standards for nursing care. Standardized nursing care plans of care or protocols also may reflect the care expected for a specific patient group. Nurses involved in setting standards should be certain the standards are realistic in light of the resources available.

If nurses do not perform duties within accepted standards of care, they may place themselves in jeopardy of legal action. In a malpractice lawsuit, these standards are used to determine whether the nurse has acted as any reasonably prudent nurse with the same level of education and experience would act. Standards of care are then guidelines for determining whether nurses performed duties in an appropriate manner. If nurses are named in malpractice lawsuits and it is shown that neither the accepted standards of care outlined by the state nursing practice act nor the policies of the employing institution were followed, the nurse's legal liability is clear.

NURSE PRACTICE ACTS AND LICENSURE

The major type of administrative law that governs nursing is licensing law. Each state has a nurse practice act, although the language of each state act is different. One aspect of the nurse-society relationship is spelled out in the state practicing act. To practice nursing, one must be licensed. This protects the consuming public from incompetent, unscrupulous, and illegal behavior.

All states have laws governing professions or occupations with general provisions for all professionals, including nursing. The nurse practice act defines nursing practice, identifies the scope of practice, outlines professional conduct, and creates a board of nursing empowered to make decisions about nursing to protect the public. Board of nursing activities include defining the scope of nursing and the entry requirements into nursing practice, such as license examinations; approving schools, faculty, curriculum, and programs in nursing; participating in disciplinary actions involving nurses; and identifying standards of care.

Specific nurse practice act provisions allow graduates of nursing programs who are waiting to take the licensure examination to practice nursing for a limited time between the time of graduation and receiving the results of the licensing examination.

THE LAW AND PRACTICE

Currently, there is pressure on the nursing profession to expand its scope of practice to new areas. When faced with such a trend, the nurses must be cognizant of the practice limitations imposed by law. Just because a patient has a need, the nurse cannot necessarily fulfill the need, if doing so requires that he or she must operate outside the scope of nursing licensure restrictions. *The prudent nurse knows the limits of practice and operates within them at all times.* Knowledge of the law, rules and regulations, and even existing institutional policy is essential to: (1) make informed decisions concerning patient care; (2) become a responsive and responsible employee in the health care system; (3) achieve personal and professional satisfaction; and (4) protect oneself from lawsuits and legal charges.

TORTS AND CRIMES

A **tort** is a wrong committed by one person against another individual or her property. The wrong is subject to action in a civil court. In most cases, a civil court will settle damages in terms of money. Torts may be intentional (assault and battery, invasion of privacy, false imprisonment, and defamation of character) or unintentional acts of wrongdoing (negligence, malpractice).

A **crime** is also a wrong against a person or his property, but the act is considered to be against the public as well. Two elements are necessary: evil intent and a criminal act. In a criminal case, the government (referred to as "The People") prosecutes the offender. When a crime is committed, the factor of intent to commit wrong is present. A crime is punished either by fines or imprisonment or both. Crimes are prosecuted in the criminal justice system and classified as felonies (e.g., rape, murder) or misdemeanors (lesser offenses generally punishable by a fine of less than $1,000 or imprisonment of less than a year).

An act generally considered a tort, because of its severity, may also be classified as a crime. For example, negligence of a gross nature that demonstrates the offender as guilty of complete disregard for another's life may be tried as both civil and criminal action. It is then prosecuted under criminal as well as civil law. By its very nature, a wrong tried as a crime implies a more serious offense with more legal implications than a tort. There are some specific laws that define the action of violators of such laws as crimes. For example, failure to observe the Federal Food,

Drug, and Cosmetic Act may constitute a crime, whether there was intent or not.

INFORMED CONSENT

Informed consent is an important aspect of the Patient's Bill of Rights. It is a person's agreement to allow something to happen (for example, surgery) based on a full exclosure of facts needed to make an intelligent decision. The facts included are the patient's current medical status and the general course of treatment; the proposed treatment and its rationale; risks and benefits of the proposed treatment; risks of not consenting to the treatment; alternatives to the proposed treatment, including nontreatment and their associated risks and benefits. All of this information must be provided to the patient in a language that he or she can understand.

Nurses have a moral obligation to ensure that patients give informed consent for their care. Health care providers are *legally* required to involve patients in health care decisions. The law has long recognized that individuals must consent to treatment. Not only must they give their consent, but they must be allowed to make an informed choice as to whether an alternative method of treatment and/or care will be provided or whether the proposed treatment is necessary. The law evolved from first demanding that physicians simply obtain permission for experimental treatment and surgery to the modern concept of giving patients full information regarding all therapeutic and diagnostic procedures.

Patients must be provided in nontechnical terms an explanation of the preferred treatment, the risks involved, alternative courses of treatment, and who will be performing the treatment or procedure. A method to ensure that patients understand what they are told should be included in these procedures.

Following such procedures not only helps avoid unnecessary lawsuits but it also establishes a relationship of trust between the patient and the health care providers. A health care provider who performs a procedure on a patient without informed consent may be found civilly liable for committing battery. It is generally the nurse's responsibility to obtain the patient's signature verifying that he or she was informed about a proposed treatment. The Joint Commission on the Accreditation of Health Organizations (JCAHO) stipulates that agencies specify in their policies which procedures require signed consent. Once a consent form is signed, the burden of proof falls to the plaintiff in a legal action against the hospital or employee.

Some states have informed consent statutes that may define the criteria for informed consent, address the need for legal competency of the patient, and stipulate who is authorized to give consent for an incompetent patient. From an ethical view, the four elements of informed consent are disclosure, voluntary choice, patient comprehension, and patient competency. Added to those elements are two variables: the right to a second opinion and the right to stop treatment any time. Competency is difficult to measure. Competency, called the capacity to make decisions, is defined as requiring possession of a set of values and goals; the ability to communicate and to understand information; and the ability to reason and to deliberate about one's choice.

A nurse and a hospital may be held liable along with a physician if there has not been adequate disclosure or other elements of informed consent have not been met. A nurse should detect a problem regarding a patient's consent when the patient does not seem to understand the procedure or risks or sign the consent form in an appropriate time period.

In any of these events, the nurse should quickly bring the situation to the attention of the physician. Also, if a patient reverses a decision and decides against treatment, the nurse is obligated to inform the physician in order to prevent unwanted treatment. Statutory and case law grant permission to administer emergency treatment without consent if it is impossible to obtain.

NEGLIGENCE AND MALPRACTICE

The standards of care that a reasonable person would use in a particular circumstance are made known through the nurse practice acts of each state, the rules and regulations established by administrative law, standard operating procedures of various health care agencies, and employee policies of the health care institution.

Deviations from the standards of care provide grounds for charges of **negligence**—the commission of an act a prudent person would not have done or the omission of a duty that a prudent person would have fulfilled, resulting in injury or harm to another person—or **malpractice**—negligence that is the proximate cause of injury resulting from a lack of professional knowledge, experience, or skill that can be expected in others in the profession.

To prove nursing malpractice, a lawyer must prove that there was a deviation from the established standard of care and that this deviation caused damage to a patient. In a malpractice case, violations of the standard of care are generally proven or disproven by expert testimony. A nurse who is an expert in a given field of nursing will frequently be called to testify about the standard of practice as it relates to that particular case.

To prove malpractice, four elements are necessary:

- A duty to the plaintiff
- A failure to meet the standard of care, or a breach of duty, which may be an act of omission
- Causation, meaning the breach of duty produced the injury in a natural and continuous sequence
- Damages, which require an actual injury to the patient

Duty describes the relationship between the plaintiff (the person bringing suit) and the defendant (the person being sued). Nurses have a duty to care for their patients. The existence of a duty is rarely an issue in a malpractice suit.

Breach of duty is the failure to conform to the standard of practice, thus creating a risk for a person that a reasonable person would have foreseen.

Although some nursing malpractice cases involve use of highly technical equipment, most cases involve assessment of routine indicators of patient well-being, such as vital signs. For example, discharging a patient with an elevated temperature, even with a written physician's order, could place the nurse in legal jeopardy. It is prudent and a reasonable standard of care that a nurse evaluate the patient's condition prior to hospital discharge and to discuss any concerns with the physician.

 ASK YOURSELF

Patient Advocacy

What should the nurse do when the physician's medical treatment does not agree with the patient's wishes and the patient is not able to participate in the decision making? If the nurse fails to speak, can he or she be held liable?

Proximate Cause

Causation must be proven for the courts to find negligence. A nurse's carelessness may not result in injury, or injury may occur without a nurse's carelessness as its proximate cause. For example, suppose a patient suffers a cardiovascular accident, and the court finds that the nurse failed to meet the standard of care because she failed to take vital signs as frequently as ordered. Is the nurse in trouble? Maybe not. The patient's paralysis may not have been directly caused by the nurse's failure to take the patient's blood pressure.

Courts frequently use foreseeability as a criterion for determining whether a cause is considered proximate cause. The question they ask is whether or not a reasonable person should have foreseen that injury as a result from failure to conform to the standard of care.

Res Ipsa Loquitur

When it is obvious that the patient's injury was the result of someone's negligence but it is impossible to prove who was at fault, the doctrine of *res ipsa loquitur* ("the thing speaks for itself") may be invoked. This principle applies when: (1) the injury could not have occurred if negligence were not present; (2) the defendant or defendants were in complete control of the instrument causing the injury; (3) the plaintiff (patient) did not voluntarily create the injury.

Damages

For a patient to prevail in a malpractice suit, the plaintiff must have suffered damages. The purpose of the suit is to compensate for these damages. *General* damages include pain and suffering, disfigurement, and disability. *Special* damages are for the losses and expenses related to the injury, such as medical expense and lost wages. *Punitive* damages are for especially malicious behavior on the part of the defendant and generally result in a larger judgment.

Liability

Liability denotes legal responsibility to pay damages. When the four elements of negligence are proven (existence of a duty, breach of duty, causation, and damages), the nurse may be found liable. The employing institution may also be held responsible for a nurse's negligence under the doctrine of *respondeat superior* ("let the master answer"). This notion of vicarious liability can be applied whenever the nurse is acting within the scope of employment. The employer may attempt to prove that the nurse was not acting within the scope of employment when the negligent act occurred. This is one reason why some nursing experts recommend that all nurses have liability insurance. Defining scope of employment is a difficult legal question, but nurses are generally covered by vicarious liability when they are acting under the control of their employer.

When a case is brought against a nurse, chances are it is a civil action that falls into one of five broad categories. These are assault, defamation of character, fraud, invasion of privacy, and false imprisonment.

Assault and Battery

Assault is the threat of touching another person without his or her consent. Battery is the actual carrying out of such a threat. The nurse may be sued for battery anytime he or she fails to obtain patient consent for a procedure.

Defamation of Character

Defamation of character includes false communication resulting in injury to a person's reputation by means of print (*libel*) or spoken word (*slander*). The nurse is permitted to make statements about a patient only as part of his or her nursing practice and only within the limits provided by the law.

Fraud

Fraud is the willful, purposeful misrepresentation of self or an act that may cause harm to a person or property. A nurse who misrepresents his or her qualifications or bills for care not given may be committing fraud.

Invasion of Privacy

The nurse is bound to limit discussion of the patient to appropriate persons. Disclosing confidential information to an inappropriate person subjects the nurse to liability for invasion of privacy, even if the information is true. The nurse may discuss the patient with others only when the discussion is necessary for treatment and care or when the patient consents to disclosure.

With the advancing use of computers in health care, many concerns are being raised by health care professionals and patient advocacy groups. Computer technology has the capability of providing charting access to patient records, individualized nursing care plans, requisitioning supplies, equipment, medications, diagnostic studies, treatment plans, scheduling and staffing, and interfacing with health care professionals across the country. Although this advancement allows for faster access to patient care and treatment information, there are significant issues surrounding confidentiality. Issues of concern include maintenance of the system's integrity, how decisions will be made regarding who should have access, data retrieval and data storage, alternatives for back-up systems in case of system failure, and should patient consent be obtained before patient information is placed in the system? Nurses need to zealously guard patient records in the Information Age.

False Imprisonment

Prevention of movement or unjustified retention of a person without consent may be false imprisonment. Nurses must use restraints only in accordance with agency policies and with the order of a physician. A patient cannot be forced to remain in the hospital against his or her will (assuming that the patient is mentally alert, oriented, and capable of participating in care decisions). If the patient refuses to remain in the hospital, the hospital will have him or her sign a release stating that he or she is leaving without medical approval. Those patients with mental impairments may be committed involuntarily in accordance with court proceedings if they are dangerous to themselves or others.

ADVANCE DIRECTIVES

The Patient Self-Determination Act (PSDA), implemented on December 1, 1991, requires all health care facilities receiving Medicare and Medicaid reimbursement to recognize the living will and durable power of attorney for health care (or health care proxy) as advance directives (Table 4–1). Though the PSDA created no new rights for patients or the public in general, it reaffirmed the common law right of self-determination as guaranteed by the Fourteenth Amendment. In addition, it requires health care facilities receiving Medicare and Medicaid funds to ask patients whether they have advance directives and to provide educational materials advising patients of their rights under existing state law.

In response to the PSDA, many health care facilities educated their staffs, created bioethics committees, and offered community education programs. On admission, each patient is asked if he or she has a living will or health care proxy, and, if so, the patient or family is asked to provide documentation. This information may be kept on file and, on

TABLE 4–1

Advance Directives Glossary

Living will (instructional directive) — allows a competent adult to give directions for future care in the event that he or she becomes incapacitated due to terminal illness or impending death. Limited to instructions given in document.

Medical power of attorney (health care proxy) — names a trusted person to act as an agent or proxy in making health care decisions in the event of incapacity. Broader implications for decision making; proxy can clarify living will or make decisions independently according to patient's values.

Prehospital advance directive specifically for Emergency Medical Services (EMS) — Depending on state or local laws, an advance directive may or may not be honored when EMS (911) is activated. For example, California, Texas, and New Jersey have enacted legislation that requires special forms to be prepared in order that EMTs not resuscitate a person.

subsequent admissions, the patient is asked to verify that these records are still valid. Documenting this process is a critical step in promoting compliance with the patient's wishes, and it may be necessary for reimbursement as well. Indeed, many hospital preadmission packets now include state-specific information about advance directives, suggested formats, and community resources that can be accessed for assistance in completing a living will or designating a health care proxy.

Of course, the usefulness of living wills may be limited to situations the individual thought about before losing the capacity to make decisions and to the clarity with which he articulated these thoughts. Health care proxies can assist in clarifying or interpreting patient wishes, but only if they have a clear sense of the patient's preferences. Many organizations provide advance directive forms that have been designed to encourage specificity and clarity and to prevent misinterpretation by others under stressful situations.

Medical and nursing literature address many factors that might influence a person's decision to write an advance directive. These include age, gender, values, economic status, educational level, and diagnosis. Researchers are now exploring the influence of cultural and ethnic values on a person's attitude toward life-sustaining treatments and tendency to complete advance directives.

The available data suggest that cultural attitudes must also be considered when approaching people and their families about end-of-life decisions. Nurses are likely to incorporate these factors into their practice because they have long been advocates of individualized care. (See Table 4–2 for Advance Directive Resources.)

In the best-case scenario, a patient, who has the support of family or significant others, presents a copy of his or her advance directive on admission and discusses its contents with his or her primary care providers. This enables the health care team to know that the document

TABLE 4–2

Advance Directive Resources for Patients

American Association of Retired Persons 601 E Street, N.W. Washington, DC 20049 (202) 434-2277	Center for Health Law and Ethics Institute of Public Law University of New Mexico School of Law 117 Stanford, N.E. Albuquerque, NM 87131 (505) 277-5006
American Bar Association 1800 M Street N.W. Washington, DC 20036 (202) 331-2297	Hastings Center Institute of Society Ethics and the Life Sciences 255 Elm Road Briarcliff Manor, NY 10510 (914) 478-0500
American Nurses Association Center for Ethics and Human Rights 600 Maryland, S.W. Suite 100W Washington, DC 20024 (800) 232-4825	Pacific Center for Health Policy and Ethics University of Southern California 444 Law Center Los Angeles, CA 90089 (213) 740-2541
Center for Bioethics of the University of Pennsylvania 3401 Market Street Suite 320 Philadelphia, PA 19104 (215) 898-7136	Local and State Offices on Aging (See your local telephone directory's White Pages)

exists, to review the patient's expressed wishes regarding his or her current condition, and to plan how caregivers should respond when providing care (Figure 4–1).

Resuscitation

The nurse must know the code status of his or her patients. The nurse verifies the code status on the patient's order sheet and follows agency policy. When nurses are unaware and encounter a patient in cardiac arrest, the patient should be resuscitated pending confirmation of a no code order. If there is a no code order, then resuscitation may be stopped once initiated.

Organ Donation

The nurse must check to see if the deceased wished to donate organs to a transplant program. If the death was accidental and no donor card is available, the nurse may discuss with the family the possibility of donating the organs of the deceased. A section of the living will may also provide this information. If functional organs are to be donated, the hospital should have specific care instructions for the body. The Uniform Anatomical Gift Act was promulgated in 1968 and adopted in all fifty states and the District of Columbia. The act was revised in 1987 and is in the process of being adopted by the states with some variation. The new act facilitates the procurement process while safeguarding donor intentions and improves procedures for use and distribution of organs (Uniform Anatomical Gift Act, 1987).

Autopsy

An autopsy is a postmortem examination of the organs and tissues of the body to determine the cause of death or the pathologic conditions contributing to the death. Consent for an autopsy is a legal requirement. The physician is responsible to request an autopsy, but family members may ask the nurse for clarification. Consent may be given by the deceased before death or by a close family member. Because of religious beliefs, some families may not consent to an autopsy, although the consent law is overruled if the death occurred because of murder or suicide, or under suspicious circumstances.

Wills

The nurse may be asked to witness a will, a person's declaration regarding how his or her property is to be handled after death. Many institutions

CONDITIONS OF ADMISSION—INPATIENT AND OUTPATIENT SERVICES

As conditions for admission for inpatient, outpatient, same day surgery or emergency treatment of the Patient whose name appears on this contract hereof, the undersigned agree as follow:

1. Consent and Treatment Authorization

The undersigned patient or other authorized representative of Patient does hereby consent to the rendering of hospital care and medical treatment which may include diagnostic testing procedures and such medical treatment and care as the attending physician and others of the Hospital medical Staff consider necessary and appropriate for the Patient's condition. Patient or Patient's authorized representative authorizes the Hospital to furnish and provide such treatment, surgical procedures, anesthesia services, x-ray examinations, laboratory and treatments, drugs, supplies, and other applications as may be ordered or requested by the attending physician or those acting in his or her place.

2. Nursing Care/Health Care Training Personnel

This hospital provides only general duty nursing care unless upon orders of the patient's physician the patient is provided more intensive nursing care. If the patient's condition is such as to need the services of a special duty nurse, it is agreed that such must be arranged by the patient or his/her legal representative. The hospital shall in no way be responsible for failure to provide the same and is hereby released from any and all liability arising from the fact that said patient is not provided with such additional care.

For the purpose of advancing the education of Health Care personnel, I hereby consent to observation and participation in my care and treatment by students enrolled in Educational Programs approved by the hospital.

3. Personal Valuables

It is understood and agreed that the hospital maintains a safe for the safekeeping of money and valuables and the hospital shall not be liable for the loss or damage to any money, jewelry, glasses, dentures, documents, furs, fur coats and fur garments or other articles of unusual value and small compass, unless placed therein, and shall not be liable for loss or damage to any other personal property, unless deposited with the hospital for safekeeping and listed on a patient valuable sheet.

6. Assignment of Insurance or Health Plan Benefits to Hospital-based Physicians

The undersigned authorizes, whether he/she signs as agent or as patient, direct payment to any Hospital-based physician of any insurance or health plan benefits otherwise payable to or on behalf of the patient for professional services rendered during this hospitalization or for outpatient services, including emergency services if rendered, at a rate not to exceed such physician's regular charges. It is agreed that payment to such physician pursuant to this authorization by an insurance company or health plan shall discharge said insurance company or health plan of any and all obligations under the policy to the extent of such payment. It is understood by the undersigned that he/she is financially responsible for charges not covered by this assignment.

7. Release of Information/Response to Inquiries

State law provides that upon an inquiry as to the presence or general condition of a specific patient, a health care facility may, unless otherwise requested by the patient, next of kin or the provider of healthcare, release at its discretion none, part of, all of, the following information: the patient's name, address, age and sex, general reason for admission, general nature of injuries or the general condition of the patient. To the extent necessary to determine the liability for payment and to obtain reimbursement, the hospital may disclose portions of the patient's records, including medical records to any person or corporation which is or may be liable for all or any portion of the hospital's charges, including but not limited to employer, insurance company, health care service plans, federal intermediaries, or workers compensation carriers.

Information may be released to insurance _____ Initials

Do not release information to insurance _____ Initials

Insurance/review organization may be contacted _____ Initials

4. Financial Agreement

The undersigned Patient and/or agent, if any, do hereby jointly and severally agree, in consideration for the rendering of services to the Patient, to pay the charges of the Hospital in accordance with the regular rates and terms of payment of the Hospital. The undersigned acknowledge that the Hospital's services are charged to the Patient and/or agent, if there is not an insurance company. The undersigned patient and/or agent, if any, accept full responsibility for charges not covered by insurance or for which payment is denied through any utilization review or pre-admission certification procedures. Should the account be referred for collection to an attorney, the undersigned agreed to pay reasonable attorneys fees and all costs of collection. All delinquent accounts bear interest at legal rate.

5. Assignment of Insurance Benefits/Medicare Patient's Release of Information

The undersigned authorizes, whether he/she signs as agent or as patient, direct payment to the Hospital of an insurance benefit otherwise payable to or on behalf of the patient for this hospitalization or for these outpatient services, including emergency services if rendered, at a rate not to exceed the Hospital's regular charge. It is agreed that payment to the Hospital pursuant to this authorization by an insurance company or health plan shall discharge said insurance company or health plan of any and all obligations under the policy to the extent of such payment. It is understood by the undersigned that he/she is financially responsible for charges not covered by this agreement.

I certify that the information given by me in applying for payment under Title XVIII of the Social Security Act is correct. I authorize release of any information needed to act on this request, and I request that payment of authorized benefits be made in my behalf. I assign payment for the unpaid charges of the physician(s) for whom the Hospital is authorized to bill in connection with its services. I understand I am responsible for any remaining balance not covered by other insurance.

8. Advanced Directive/Patient Rights Information

A. I have been informed of my rights to formulate Advance Directives

☐ Yes ☐ No
_____
Initials

B. I have been given written materials about my right to accept or refuse medical treatment

☐ Yes ☐ No
_____
Initials

Patient brochure given? ☐ Yes

9. Community Memorial is a Non-Smoking Facility

10. The undersigned certifies that he/she has read the foregoing, receiving a copy thereof, and is the patient, or is duly authorized by the patient as patient's general agent to execute the above and accept its terms.

Patient's Signature: _____

Date: _____   Time: _____

Other: _____

_____ / _____
Name   Relationship

Date: _____   Time: _____

Witness: _____
                        Hospital Representative

Date: _____   Time: _____

FIGURE 4–1 Conditions of admission. *Reprinted with permission of Community Memorial Hospital.*

have policies about nurses witnessing legal documents. If a nurse witnesses a will, the nurse makes a note on the patient's chart about the patient's mental and physical condition at the time of the signing and of the nurse's role in the procedures. A nurse cannot be a beneficiary to any will he or she witnesses.

Refusal of Treatment

The patient has a right to refuse treatment. Refusal of treatment often involves complex issues such as refusal of blood transfusions for religious reasons or the predetermined decisions regarding refusal to initiate or maintain life-sustaining measures. Problems also frequently arise with emotional decisions that family members make for care of minor children or for care of incompetent parents. Dealing with these complex issues calls for accurate documentation of the patient's condition, level of consciousness, and verbatim expression of the patient's intent and rationale. In many health care facilities an ethics committee composed of physicians, nurses, clergy, attorneys, psychologists, and ethicists is available to make recommendations regarding individual cases of actual or potential refusal of life-sustaining treatment. A signed release of liability such as a hospital's discharge "against medical advice" is evidence that the patient refused treatment or recommended care.

PRIVACY

In an increasingly consumer-oriented society, patients are becoming more interested in learning details about the services they receive and the rationale for those services. Although a health care organization's records belong to the organization, confidential information in a record is accessible by right only to the patient to whom it belongs. Because the record is confidential, the patient or legal guardian must sign a release of information whenever a record or portion thereof will be reviewed outside of direct caregivers of the organization. Release of this information should not be a general release but should specifically state what part of the clinical record or what topic of information is to be released and to whom.

If a health care organization receives patient information or documents from another organization, the second organization may not release the forms to a third party without the first organization's documented approval. Usually, the patient would need to sign another release form from the first agency, documenting specifically to whom the information would be released. For the same reason, telephone calls between health care professionals should be handled with confidentiality of information in mind. No information should be given unless a patient authorizes the release in writing (Figure 4–2).

Patients have the right to view their own clinical record. Some safeguards, however, are advisable. When a patient or family member views the medical record, a nurse or physician should be in attendance to explain terminology, phrases, or rationales.

Health care organizations have specific policies and procedural guidelines for health care professionals to follow if a patient requests to see his or her chart. The procedures may include notification of the department or unit manager or supervisor, the risk management department representative, the administrative supervisor on duty or on call, the physician, and the social services department representative. Various organizations will have various persons and/or departments to notify when this issue arises. Nursing documentation should be written with the idea that the patient does have right of access to the record.

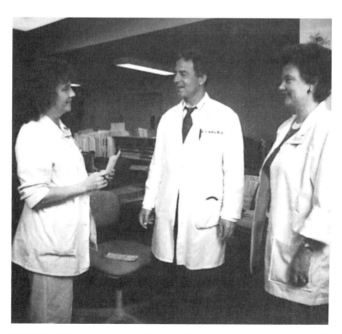

FIGURE 4-2 Nurses and other health care professionals should not discuss patients, families, or coworkers in public areas.

ADDITIONAL AREAS OF CONCERN

There are several additional aspects of a nurse's job that are a potential for legal liability. These include verbal orders, incidents such as falls, and the use of restraints.

Verbal Orders

Verbal orders are medical orders from the physician when the physician is communicating orally, most often by telephone. The purpose of the verbal order is to provide for continuity and update of care according to the patient's needs when the physician is not available to submit written orders. A well-written verbal order should document that it is not an on-site order. The nurse taking the verbal order should document the order, his or her name, the date and time the order was taken, and the time the order is being written and transcribed. Following is an example:

> 1-13-90, 3:00 P.M. Verbal order received by telephone from Dr. Maxwell Jones for Mrs. Joanna Stephens, d/c IV after last ordered bag.

The verbal order should be signed by the physician within 24 hours in acute care settings. An unsigned medical order can be flagged in the chart to remind the physician that an order needs his or her signature. In home health care, the verbal order should be signed by the physician within 8 days. In this setting, the verbal order may be mailed to the physician for signature and returned to the home health agency. Facsimile machines and computer networks facilitate this procedure.

A significant problem with verbal orders is the potential for error. After repeating the verbal order to the physician, the nurse has a legal and ethical obligation to question and/or challenge questionable orders. (This obligation also refers to written orders.) It is prudent for the nurse to seek information, clarification, and satisfaction before documenting and executing a medical order.

Falls

Ethical and legal guidelines indicate that hospitals have a duty to take reasonable precautions to provide safety to patients who are likely to injure themselves. Nursing facilities have taken the lead in developing organized alert systems to identify elderly residents who have potential to fall or have fallen recently. In some organizations, ribbons or stickers are used to identify patients likely to fall by placing these indicators on the door, chart, bed, and wheelchair or walker.

Risk assessments are done routinely, and all workers from supervisor to staff nurse are to observe and assist in preventing falls. Recent research has identified the following significant risk factors for falls: decreased level of mobility; three or more medical diagnoses, especially cardiovascular or musculoskeletal disease; use of three or more drugs daily, particularly cardiovascular, antihypertensive, tranquilizer, or antidepressant drugs.

Documentation in the patient record should include an assessment of a patient's level of consciousness, balance, and mobility as well as precautions taken to prevent falls by assistance or restraints. Further, documentation should also include any declarations of intentions to assist a patient made by family members or other caregivers, and the responsibilities each had agreed to accept in care of the patient.

Restraints

Accidents and injuries occur even when a patient is restrained. Physical and chemical restraints impose an obligation on the nurse to carefully and frequently monitor a patient's condition. Restraints should be used judiciously and according to the health care organization's policy and procedure and always with a physician's order. Restrained arms and legs should be assessed routinely for circulation and skin condition and release from restraints should allow periodic, routine exercise.

Nursing documentation should reflect patient observations. Documented actions should reflect state law and health care organization standards regarding restraints—their application, duration, and frequency of observation. It should also include the reasons the patient is restrained, what method of restraint is used, the patient's response, outcome, safety, and assessment of the continued need for restraint.

Long-term care facilities, in accordance with federal and state laws, have developed stringent policies regarding the use of physical and chemical restraints on patients. Using clinical judgment to decrease physical and chemical restraints is closely related to potential for injury assessments and risk management.

In the long-term care setting, physical restraints refer to the use of straps or safety vests to maintain a patient's position in bed or in a chair. Virtually all health care providers believe that it is essential for patients to maintain dignity and independence by permitting them to take "normal risks of daily living." Restraints used in an attempt to remove these normal risks violate the rights of patients, reduce their quality of life, and present significant physical and psychological risks. Restraints used at a long-term care facility are considered to treat the medical symptom or condition that endangers the physical safety of the patient or other patients and under the following conditions: (1) as a last resort measure after a trial period where less restrictive measures have been undertaken and proven unsuccessful; (2) with physician order; (3) with the consent of the patient (or legal representative); (4) when the benefits of the restraints outweigh the identified risks.

Patients are assessed at admission and periodically throughout residency at a long-term care facility. Assessments include the reason for the restraints, if the patient can safely and independently get out of a chair, whether the patient has fallen within the past 6 months, and whether the patient is receiving any medication that affects balance or alertness. When restraints are needed, the least restrictive type for the shortest period of time is implemented.

Information is carefully documented in the chart for clinical judgment to initiate restraints and for documentation support for continued restraint use. Documentation of assessment, frequent reassessment, intervention, and patient response to restraints is important because this is a high-risk area of care in all health care settings.

INCIDENT REPORTS

Any unusual occurrence in hospital routine or in patient care should be documented. The occurrence may have resulted in an actual injury to a patient (or employee or visitor) or a situation that may potentially cause injury. This report can be used for any injury, errors in treatment or medication administration, or loss or damage to a patient, nurse, or organization's property. Falls, burns, and medication errors are the most common incidents in a hospital. Nurses have a contractual responsibility to complete incident reports for any incident in which they are involved. Furthermore, insurance companies often have the contractual policy with a health care organization that unless they are given an incident report in a timely manner regarding the incident, they will not insure the resulting litigation expenses.

For legal reasons, the existence of the incident report should not be mentioned in nursing documentation in the chart. These reports should not be attached to the chart. This procedure assists the health care organization in keeping the information nondiscoverable from attorneys for the potential plaintiff (the suing patient) (Figure 4–3).

The incident report is an internal device for the health care organization. It is considered necessary for the internal use in the quality assurance program and is only available on a confidential basis to the committee during quality assurance meetings. Under these conditions, the incident report is deemed privileged information, which prevents its release to a plaintiff's attorneys.

The patient's condition before the accident or injury is an important focus of information, especially as it relates to the possible cause of the injury. Any action the patient engaged in or any refusal of medical or nursing direction before the incident should be documented if it appears that patient behavior contributed to the incident. For example, documentation in the nurse's notes before a fall states a nurse instructed the patient to call for help with the call bell that the nurse put within reach. This information can be repeated on the incident report. If the patient sues, a judge or jury may determine that the patient contributed to the injury by not following the nurse's direction. Therefore, the nurse and the hospital would not be liable.

A second focus of information is the condition of the patient after the incident. Assessment should be thorough, concise, and focused on objective and subjective signs and symptoms related to the site(s) of actual injury or potential injury. Absence of pertinent symptoms or complaints of pain are important to document. In an incident in which a patient fell and injured one knee, the assessment portion of the note might read: "R knee slightly red, no induration, skin intact. Pt has full ROM of joint without complaint of pain. Able to continue ambulation with no pain per patient."

A third important focus of information is the nursing intervention after the incident. After a fall in which a patient complains of pain in her upper arm, for example, documentation could read: "Pt assisted back to bed. Skin and ROM of R upper arm inspected, vital signs checked, assessed situation precipitating fall, reinstructed patient to prevent further incidents."

The first page of the incident report is completed by the nurse who was in attendance during an incident or who first saw the patient after an incident. If a nurse is not in attendance when an incident or accident occurs, the nurse's documentation must clearly show the patient was found after the accident. For example, a nurse found a patient sitting on the floor and the patient stated she fell trying to walk to the bedside commode.

Do not Photocopy

NOTIFICATION FORM
THIS REPORT IS CONFIDENTIAL—
NOT A PART OF THE MEDICAL RECORD

Section I
If no addressograph plate, complete the following two (2) items:

_____
Name of Patient or Person Involved

_____
Medical Record or other Identification Number

_____
Print name of person completing this form

_____
Location or Cost Center

Section II

SEX: M F (Circle one)

Check One:
☐ Outpatient/ER   ☐ Inpatient
☐ Visitor   ☐ Volunteer

AGE [____] If Under 1 Year, circle one:
0–14 days   15–364 days

DATE OF OCCURRENCE ___ / ___ / ___
                    MM   DD   YY

TIME OF OCCURRENCE _____ AM PM
                            (circle one)

Section III (When checked, omit AA-B-C-D)

A.   1.00 ☐ Patient's property missing or damaged

AA. 1.20 ☐ Return of a patient to the Operating Room
     1.40 ☐ Newborn problem

Check ONE box in EACH of the following groups.

B.   EVENT HAPPENING DURING THIS ADMISSION
     2.00   ☐ Not applicable or Unknown
     2.10   ☐ Consent for Procedure
     2.20   ☐ Diet

DESCRIPTION OF OCCURRENCE— *Briefly* describe what happened. Name the equipment, drug, treatment, or procedure, etc., involved, and parts of the body affected. DO NOT mention names of individuals in this section: _____

_____
_____
_____
_____
_____
_____

THIS SECTION FOR ADMINISTRATIVE USE ONLY

MEDICATION:
☐ Omission   ☐ Incorrect Time
☐ Incorrect Dose   ☐ Incorrect Drug
☐ Incorrect Route ☐ Unordered Drug
☐ Extra Dose   ☐ Narcotic Drug
☐ Adverse Reaction ☐ Transcription Error

NURSE:

☐ RN I   ☐ RN II   ☐ LVN   ☐ FLOAT

☐ Other _____

SEVERITY RATING:

☐ Level 0   No medication error occurred (potential error).

☐ Level 1   An error occurred that did not result in patient harm.

☐ Level 2   An error occurred that resulted in the need for increased patient monitoring, but no change in vital signs and no patient harm.

☐ Level 3   An error occurred that resulted in the need for increased monitoring, with a change in vital signs, but no harm done.
      • OR needed increased lab studies monitoring (glucose, PTT)

☐ Level 4   An error occurred that resulted in the need for treatment with another drug, or an increased length of stay or that affected patient participation in an investigational drug study.

☐ Level 5   An error occurred that resulted in permanent or severe patient harm.

☐ Level 6   An error occurred that resulted in patient death.

2.30 ☐	AMA or Elopement
2.31 ☐	Out of Bed or Unit
2.35 ☐	Equipment or Medical Device
2.40 ☐	I.V. Infusion
2.50 ☐	Fall Unattended
2.51 ☐	Fall Attended
2.60 ☐	Fire
2.70 ☐	Medication
2.80 ☐	Transfusion
2.90 ☐	Treatment or Procedure
2.95 ☐	Other

C. EFFECT HAPPENING DURING THIS ADMISSION

3.00 ☐	No Apparent Effect
3.10 ☐	Aspiration—Foreign Matter
3.15 ☐	Burn
3.20 ☐	Cardiac Arrest
3.21 ☐	Myocardial Infarction
3.25 ☐	Decubitus Ulcer
3.30 ☐	Drug Reaction or Toxic Effect
3.35 ☐	Fracture
3.40 ☐	Infection
3.45 ☐	Laceration
3.46 ☐	Bruise, Abrasion, Contusion
3.50 ☐	Neurological Impairment
3.55 ☐	Hemorrhage
3.60 ☐	Pulmonary Embolism
3.65 ☐	Retained Foreign Body
3.70 ☐	Vascular Impairment of an Extremity
3.75 ☐	Wound Disruption
3.95 ☐	Any Other Effect _____

D. SEVERITY OF EFFECT

4.10 ☐	Effect Nonexistent or Unknown
4.20 ☐	Effect Inconsequential
4.30 ☐	Effect Consequential
4.40 ☐	Death

FIGURE 4–3 Incident report. *Reprinted with permission of Community Memorial Hospital.*

continues

1.20   Return of the patient to the operating room during this admission
1.40   Newborn problems include one or more of the following: coma, convulsions, Apgar less than 5 at 5 minutes, or gestation less than 35 weeks.

Event is a happening which is not consistent with the routine care and treatment related to the patient's admitting or working diagnosis.

An event may involve any one of the following:

Which may have arisen out of one of the following:

A. Prescription out of order
B. Method of administration or performance
C. Omission
D. Misidentification of amount or dose
E. Misidentification of drug, substance, or treatment
F. Misidentification of patient
G. Contamination
H. Malfunction

2.10   Consent for Procedure
2.20   Diet
2.31   Out of Bed or Unit
2.35   Equipment or Medical Device
2.40   I.V. Infusion
2.70   Medication
2.80   Transfusion
2.90   Treatment/Procedure

2.30   AMA or Elopement   }
2.50   Fall Unattended   }   All AMA's, elopements, falls, and fires are subject to notification
2.51   Fall Attended   }
2.60   Fire   }

Effect is a temporary or permanent impairment of physical or mental function which is not an intended result of the care and treatment related to the patient's admitting or working diagnosis.

An Effect may be one of the following:

3.10   *Aspiration of foreign matter* into the respiratory tract.
3.15   *Burn* of any tissue, internal or external.
3.20   *Cardiac arrest* whenever resuscitation attempted.
3.21   *Myocardial infarction* not present on admission.
3.25   *Decubitus ulcer* in any location.
3.30   *Drug reaction or toxic effect*, immediate or delayed.

3.35   *Fracture*, displaced or undisplaced.
3.40   *Infection* of any wound or organ not present on admission to hospital.
3.45   *Laceration* of skin or any structure, internal or external.
3.46   *Bruise*, *Abrasion*, *Contusion* not present on admission.
3.50   *Neurological impairment*, central or peripheral, not present on admission, such as convulsions, coma, loss of taste, sight, hearing, numbness, weakness, and paralysis.
3.60   *Pulmonary embolism* from any source.
3.65   *Retained foreign body*, not intended.
3.70   *Vascular impairment of an extremity* involving arteries or veins.
3.75   *Wound disruption*, with or without evisceration of internal organs; may involve internal or external wound or anastamosis.

Severity of Effect

4.20   Inconsequential: A transient, nondisabling impairment, not requiring surgical correction, narcotic analgesia antibiotic therapy, not requiring new management nor a probable increase in length of stay.

4.30   Consequential: Impairment requiring a new management or a probable increased length of stay.

WITNESS   Name _____   Name _____

Address _____   Address _____

Phone # _____   Phone # _____

FIGURE 4–3 *continued*

The nurse does not document that the patient fell because the nurse did not see the fall. He or she only documents the condition of the patient when first observed after the accident. The nurse assesses and documents the patient's condition and complaints of pain and documents the patient's statement regarding how the accident occurred. Also the nurse documents any interventions the nurse performed after the incident and to whom the incident was reported.

The second page of the incident report allows additional documentation of a witness's objective description of an incident. The space may also be used to document additional statements made to the nursing supervisor at the time of the incident or after the incident by the patient or other caregivers.

Writing incident reports may seem time consuming and pointless. Some nurses even try to avoid writing incident reports; however, these reports are actually helpful in defense of nurses, as a protection of rights for patients, and as tools to improve quality of care. Every nurse should conscientiously fill out incident reports.

THE LEGAL PROCESS

Litigation (a lawsuit) begins when a complaining party (the plaintiff) files a document known as a complaint (pleading made by a plaintiff under oath to initiate a lawsuit) with the court. This document states the basis for the complaint and outlines the damages (money asked for by the plaintiff as compensation for any loss, detriment, or injury to the plaintiff's person, property, or rights caused by the wrongdoing or negligence of the defendant). The person at whom the complaint is directed is known as the defendant. The filing of a complaint is followed by the issue of a summons, which is a court order advising the defendant that a lawsuit against him or her is pending. It further notifies the defendant what he or she must do with respect to the lawsuit and the time constraints involved.

A defendant presented with a summons normally retains an attorney, who then files a document called an appearance, which prevents the court from entering a default judgment. The defendant, through his attorney, then files a response (answer) to the allegations made in the complaint. This response either admits or denies the allegations made. If the response by the defendant includes significant information not referred to in the original complaint, the plaintiff, through his attorney, has the option to file a reply. If the defendant, once served, chooses to do nothing in response to the summons, such as hire an attorney or file a counter complaint, the court may enter a default judgment against the defendant, which is based on the uncontested testimony of the plaintiff. See Table 4–3 for various reasons for patient litigation.

When all the allegations by both parties have been addressed, the case is ready to move forward and the parties are said to be "at issue." Discovery procedures (pretrial procedures allowing one party to examine vital witnesses and/or documents held exclusively by the adverse party) are then initiated, whereby relevant information is gathered by both sides. Depositions (out-of-court, under oath statements of a witness) and interrogatories (written questions) are taken from or asked of witnesses before the scheduled trial. During this pretrial period, efforts may be made by either side to influence the outcome of the lawsuit. Such efforts include, but are not limited to, motions to dismiss the complaint, requests to change the trial date, and offers of a settlement out of court.

If motions to dismiss the lawsuit are denied and all other motions have been resolved by the court, the case then goes to trial. The court hears the evidence, comes to certain conclusions, and decides on a verdict. Once the judge or jury reaches a decision and a verdict is declared, either party may appeal (request review and/or retrial of legal issues) that verdict to an appellate court. If an appeal is granted, the testimony and the procedures of the trial are reviewed by the appellate court. That court may choose to uphold or reverse the decision of the lower court.

TABLE 4–3

Common Reasons for Patient Litigation

- Improper use of equipment or supplies
- Inappropriate performance of a procedure
- Failure to follow a physician's order correctly and in a timely manner
- Lack of protection from falls and other injuries
- Lack of appropriate patient observation and monitoring
- Failure to function within area of expertise
- Inappropriate administration of medications
- Unexpected change in patient's condition or treatment outcome
- Loss of rapport or poor rapport with hospital
- Inappropriate or lack of patient education

The right to an appeal is a constitutional right and serves as part of the system of checks and balances on the court system of the United States.

The time period for the process of litigation and the outcome of that litigation vary, depending on many factors that are peculiar to each case. Predominant factors are (1) the severity of the complaint, (2) whether an injury or a death is involved, and (3) the backlog of cases pending before the court.

MALPRACTICE INSURANCE

In the section on liability, the doctrine of *respondeat superior* was discussed. Vicarious liability may be applied whenever the nurse is acting within the scope of employment. Nurses who support the idea of vicarious liability believe that individual malpractice insurance is not necessary. They are therefore reluctant to purchase their own malpractice insurance.

No one want to be sued, or be forced into court. Yet, the fact of the matter is that nurses are all too often required to appear in court to defend themselves. Many nurses feel that malpractice insurance is the only answer.

The employer, in a litigation, may attempt to prove that the nurse was not acting within the scope of employment when the negligent act occurred. This is one of the primary reasons that some nursing experts believe that all nurses should have individual malpractice insurance. Additionally, if the nurse and the employer are co-defendants and are found liable, and if the settlement costs are more than the employer's policy provides, the nurse may be required to pay the difference. Furthermore, there is also the argument that the health care agency's attorney(s) will be representing the agency and protecting the agency's

---

 ASK YOURSELF

Legal Practice

How are you protecting yourself from potential lawsuits? Are you practicing nursing according to established standards of care? Why does the number of lawsuits involving nurses continue to increase? What role does nursing education play in developing guidelines to reduce the number of lawsuits?

interests, not the nurse's. The employer's insurance company may sue the nurse if the company believes that, because of the nurse's action, they have suffered a loss. Whatever the preference, nurses should investigate insurance policies carefully.

Some health care agencies carry liability insurance for the employer and the employee. Based on the limitations of the policy, liability insurance may cover the costs of legal counsel and provide protection in the case of judgment or settlement.

Nurses may obtain liability insurance from several companies and through various professional organizations. Many companies advertise through professional magazines, and the application for membership is often included with the advertisement. Mass marketing has been effective in helping to keep the premiums for nurses' liability insurance at a reasonable cost. See Table 4-4 for guidelines to reduce risks of litigation.

How much insurance coverage should a nurse purchase? It is a difficult question at best. Some insurance carriers no longer offer a $500,000 policy because of the larger settlements now being awarded and they report that nurses are requesting $1,000,000 to $1,500,000 policies. The costs can range from $75 to $150 per year. Nurses should do comparative evaluations of policies before purchasing to be assured of getting the best coverage for their particular area of practice. Some advance practice nurses such as nurse midwives, nurse anesthetists, and nurse practitioners are required to pay increased costs for their liability insurance.

Comparison shopping is a must for the nurse before purchasing liability coverage. Most companies are receptive to providing brochures

TABLE 4-4

Guidelines for Reducing Risk of Litigation

- Know your scope of practice.
- Be familiar with the agency's policies and procedures.
- Chart objectively, timely, accurately, and completely.
- Remain current in nursing practice.
- Establish and maintain rapport with patients and families.
- Be involved in nursing practice evaluation.
- Question unclear or ambiguous physician orders.
- Monitor patients for responses to treatments and procedures.
- Take special precautions with verbal orders.

and copies of the policy for review and evaluation. It is well worth the time investment to find the company that provides the coverage for the best protection.

There is variety in malpractice policies for nurses although the basics are similar. For example, a liability policy may include personal liability coverage, which means that the nurse may be covered for non-nursing incidents. When evaluating policies, the questions in Table 4–5 may be used to help in making decisions about appropriate coverage.

Liability policies should be read carefully to make certain that all issues are understood. Other important items to remember are: (1) if the nurse changes a position or status, the insurer should be notified in writing; (2) keep a copy of all written notifications to the insurer and all written notices from the insurer; written correspondence should include the nurse's name and policy number; (3) the insurer should be notified of any incidents involving the nurse that may lead to litigation;

TABLE 4–5

Evaluating Malpractice Insurance

- What are the financial limitations of the policy?
- Who is covered?
- Under what conditions is the policy renewable?
- What is the annual premium cost?
- How long does the coverage last? (Occurrence coverage refers to coverage for any incidents that occurred while the policy was in effect, even if a suit is filed after a policy has lapsed. Claims-made-coverage means that coverage is provided only if the claim is filed while the policy is in effect.)
- When am I covered? On the job and off the job?
- Am I provided with an attorney? This does not mean that you get to choose the attorney or to decide when you need one. The insurance company may make those decisions, depending on your policy coverage.
- Is my salary guaranteed when I am in court?
- Am I required to settle?
- What other items are included in the coverage?
- Is there a limit on the number of cases covered in a specific time period?

(4) the nurse may call the company about an incident or issue that needs clarification; (5) all telephone calls to the insurance company should include the nurse's name and policy number for correct identification, the name of the person the nurse spoke with, what was said, and the date and time of conversation.

When canceling the policy, it is important to follow the policy guideline and rules for the procedure. Most insurers require the nurse to return the policy and notify the company by letter, with the date the coverage is to end.

GOOD SAMARITAN LAW

The Good Samaritan law offers legal immunity for health care professionals who assist in an emergency and render reasonable care under such circumstances. Because most states do not require nurses or citizens to aid the distressed, such assistance becomes an ethical, rather than a legal duty. Although this law limits liability for the nurse, he or she may be liable for gross negligence. A nurse who stops to help is obligated to remain until additional assistance is obtained. The nurse should then relinquish care to official rescue personnel unless asked to remain. Because emergency assistance is generally outside the scope of the nurse's employment, the employer's malpractice insurance will not provide coverage. This is another reason why many nursing legal experts say that nurses should carry their own malpractice insurance.

PROTECTING YOURSELF AND DOCUMENTATION

Nurses can minimize the risk of legal problems, including malpractice, in a number of ways. First, nurses must keep current with advances in clinical nursing practice. Continuing education is absolutely essential to stay knowledgeable regarding general and particular expectations of nurses. Likewise, nurses should be familiar with state regulations governing nursing and with standards of professional organizations.

Nurses involved in the development of policies, procedures, protocols, or standardized nursing plans of care should be sure to make them realistic, whether for home or an agency. Such measures of the standard of care should not be made unless they can be applied with the resources available. Staffing and equipment to conform to these guidelines must be available on nights, weekends, holidays, and weekdays. Those who develop standards to apply to various practice settings should keep in mind the differences in resources and facilities of different sizes, acuity, and geographic area. Those involved in policy making need to continue to update the policies to be timely and sensible in accordance with the demands of nursing. New knowledge based on sound research must be applied. Policies, procedures, and protocols must be followed. Propounding unrealistic policies and procedures that are not followed is an invitation to malpractice suits.

The condition of the patient must be monitored and the observations documented. Whether the patient is in a hospital recovering from surgery, in home care coping with a chronic illness, or dealing with long-term, multiple drug administration, assessment of the patient must be recorded. Significant changes in the patient's condition need to be reported to the physician in a timely manner. The report to the physician also must be documented. When physicians do not follow up with assessment intervention, their care needs to be challenged by the nurse. Hospitals may be liable when nurses do not challenge physicians in the face of obvious negligence.

Documentation should be accurate, complete, and contemporaneous with the care given. Documentation should include normal findings in the form of a flow sheet, checklist, or narrative. When critical events occur, the precise time should be noted in the records. Vital signs need to be assessed in accordance with agency policy and recorded. Documentation should be objective. Criticism of other providers does not belong in the medical record. Negative comments about the patient or family should not be included in the medical record, unless they constitute objective documentation of behavior or accurate quotations of statements made. Errors should be corrected by marking a line through the error and recording the nurse's initials. An entry should never be obliterated. The presumption will be that the matter erased is more damaging than whatever was actually written. If a specific incident, such as a fall or medication error, occurs, follow these principles:

- Maintain rapport with the patient. Do not avoid communication with the patient who is experiencing stress and uncertainty. Offer simple explanations if you can do so honestly, calmly, and without blaming anyone.
- Document the incident in the progress notes and the appropriate forms used by your institution. Incident reports are useful to

remind you of the events surrounding an incident, and they are useful to bring about needed changes in the institution.

Nursing standards of care outline and define appropriate nursing interventions. Some standards are stated in general terms such as those enacted in nursing practice acts and those provided by professional nursing organizations. More specific standards are defined by the employing institutions. If nurses act within the accepted standard of care, their chances of being involved in a malpractice lawsuit are reduced.

Some legal issues, such as the necessity for informed consent and avoiding negligence, are involved in almost every branch of nursing. *Nurses are responsible for knowing the laws that apply to their areas of nursing practice.*

KEY POINTS

- In negligence and malpractice cases, four elements decide the merits of a case: legal duty, breach of duty, proximate cause, and damage.
- Law and ethics together influence behavior. Law and ethics are two forces that help people ensure rights, minimize potential harm, and guide human behavior. Laws are mandatory guidelines people must follow under obligation of fines or incarceration.
- Nurses are potentially subject to discipline by the licensing authority when malpractice occurs, which involves care below the standard of care or when care rendered is beyond the scope of nursing practice.
- Although the Good Samaritan law provides immunity for professionals under specific circumstances, it will not protect the nurse who is negligent in his or her practice.
- One way to avoid malpractice litigation is to follow the current standard of nursing care as evidenced in state statutes and regulations, standards of professional organizations, and current literature.
- When documentation follows policies and procedures and is written with legal issues in mind, the law can protect nurses and health care organizations from charges of negligence and malpractice.

CRITICAL THINKING ACTIVITIES

1. As a class assignment, your nursing class study group is asked to prepare a presentation on advance directives to be presented to a 50+ seniors group at one of the local acute hospital clinical sites. Design an outline of the subjects to be included in the presentation. Provide a list of resources for additional information as a handout for the group.

2. What are the legal considerations for nurses involved in patient care situations involving pronouncement of death and do not resuscitate orders?

3. If as a nurse you accept a fee for the services rendered during an emergency situation, are there legal implications for accepting compensation for your professional nursing services? Would you be protected by the Good Samaritan Act?

CASE STUDY

During your home health nursing experience, you see a patient who is 70 years old, lives alone, and has chronic obstructive pulmonary disease. During your visits, you note that the patient is growing weaker, more fatigued, struggling with shortness of breath, and during the last month he has lost approximately 10 lbs. He has three adult children who live in the local area and they each take turns transporting him to his clinic and physician appointments. One of his daughters is concerned about her father's condition and the increasing amount of care he requires. She mentions her concerns to you. You know that patients with this disease deteriorate with time, and they often require ventilator support when they no longer have the strength to breathe on their own.

1. Design assessments of the patient's and family's comprehension and expectations of the patient's deteriorating health.

2. Based on those data, identify planning and interventions that you believe are needed. Identify patient and family teaching and the appropriate teaching strategies.

3. Propose additional information you need to supply the family, so you can assist them in planning realistic possibilities for the future.

⇒ CASE STUDY

As a licensed nurse, you are one of two team leaders working the evening shift on a busy medical-surgical unit in a metropolitan hospital. The other team leader is also the nurse in charge for the shift. Several of the patients in your colleague's team have repeatedly requested pain medication During his lunch break, one of the patients states that she is going to ask her family to telephone her physician because she can't seem to get any pain relief from her current medication being administered for pain.

You have worked with this nurse several times during the past few months and you have noticed similar complaints from other patients. You have some concerns about appropriate patient care and you decide that some action should be taken. Who should you speak with first, the nursing colleague or the supervisor of the unit? Write what you plan to say to either person. What are your thoughts supporting your statements or questions? Depending on who you talk with, what are the risks? What should your plan of action be? What resources are available to provide assistance?

BIBLIOGRAPHY

Aiken, T. (1994). *Legal issues in nursing*. Philadelphia: Addison-Wesley.

Barnett, C. (1995). Legal questions. *Nursing 95, 25*(5), 30–32.

Bosna, M. (1995). Legal questions. *Nursing 95, 25*(70), 71–73.

Creighton, H. (1986). *Law every nurse should know* (5th ed). Philadelphia: W. B. Saunders

Fiesta, J. (1995). Legal aspects—Standards of care: Part I. *Nursing Management, 24*(70), 31.

Hogstel, M. O. (1994). *Nursing care of the older adult* (3rd ed.). Albany, NY: Delmar Publishers.

Kolodner, D. (1993). Preventing malpractice. *Medsurg Nursing, 2*(5), 405.

Roach, W. (1994). *Medical records and the law* (2nd ed.). Gaithersburg, MD: Aspen.

Shea, M. A. (1996). When a patient refuses treatment. *RN, 59*(7), 51–54.

INTERNET RESOURCES

Centers for Disease Control and Prevention
   http://www.cdc/gov
Department of Health and Human Services
   http://www.os.dhhs.gov
Food and Drug Administration
   http://www.fda.gov
Health Care Financing Administration
   http://www.hcfa.gov
Joint Commission on the Accreditation of Healthcare Organizations
   http://www.jcaho.org
National Institutes of Health
   http://www.nih.gov
Social Security Administration
   http://www.ssa.gov
U.S. federal government agencies
   http://www.lib.lsu.edu/gov/fedgov.html
Veterans Administration
   http://www.va.gov

CHAPTER 5

Ethical Nursing Practice

OVERVIEW

A code of ethics, basic to all professions, groups, and cultures, consist of rules or guidelines concerned with appropriate conduct and actions. Ethical codes *or* codes of ethics represent judgments about moral responsibility and obligations. This chapter is in some respects a discussion of the essential nursing values and nursing accountability. The principles of ethics are presented, including ethical theory frameworks. The presentation on principles focuses on the principle-based approach and the care-based approach to health care. Current ethical issues in nursing are also addressed, including staffing shortages and nurse incompetence.

OBJECTIVES

Upon completion of this chapter, the reader should be able to:

- Define values and explain accountability as it relates to ethical behavior.
- Describe the common modes of values transmission.
- Discuss two theory frameworks and their relationship to ethical decision making.
- Define the four major principles of health care ethics.
- Explain case analysis in making ethical decisions.
- Discuss specific ethical issues in nursing as presented.

⮞ **KEY TERMS**

Advance directive	Fidelity
Advocacy	Justice
Autonomy	Nonmaleficence
Beneficence	Veracity
Confidentiality	

INTRODUCTION

Members of professions have specialized knowledge and expertise that are used to make critical decisions. Often these decisions affect the lives of other people. The purpose of a code of ethics is to describe the correct and moral way to use this power. In nursing, ethics provide standards for professional activities, which protect both nurse and patient.

Concerns about right and wrong are not new, but today's society is changing more rapidly than in the past. Advances in medical knowledge and technology, together with societal and political changes, are raising a number of well-publicized moral dilemmas for both patients and health care professionals. Less well-publicized, but no less important, are the troubling conflicts of values that arise for nurses in these changing circumstances. Many of the concerns are emotionally charged and require intensive debate and discussion. See the Patient's Bill of Rights in Table 5–1.

There is often conflict in values, problem resolution, professional judgment, and professional options. To resolve potential conflicts many professions—such as nursing—are governed by a definite framework. This establishes various rules and roles that provide unambiguous direction. Although a framework works well for simple issues, in very complex matters, nurses must consider all aspects of an issue and know what their rights are, as well as the rights of the patient. Additionally, professional values are shaped by personal values. Nurses need to examine their intuitions, opinions, and convictions about what is morally right or wrong and monitor how they influence their nursing care.

TABLE 5–1

The Patient's Bill of Rights

- The patient has the right to considerate and respectful care.

- The patient has the right to obtain from his physician complete current information concerning his diagnosis, treatment, and prognosis in terms the patient can be reasonably expected to understand. When it is not medically advisable to give such information to the patient, the information should be made available to an appropriate person in his behalf. He has the right to know, by name, the physician responsible for coordinating his care.

- The patient has the right to receive from his physician information necessary to give informed consent prior to the start of any procedure and/or treatment. Except in emergencies, such information for informed consent should include, but not necessarily be limited to, the specific procedure and/or treatment, the medically significant risks involved, and the probable duration of incapacity. Where medically significant alternatives for care or treatment exist, or when the patient requests information concerning medical alternatives, the patient has the right to such information. The patient also has the right to know the name of the person responsible for the procedures and/or treatment.

- The patient has the right to refuse treatment to the extent permitted by law, and to be informed of the medical consequences of his action.

- The patient has the right to every consideration of his privacy concerning his own medial care program. Case discussion, consultation, examination, and treatment are confidential and should be conducted discreetly. Those not involved in his care must have permission of the patient to be present.

- The patient has the right to expect that all communications and records pertaining to his care should be treated as confidential.

- The patient has the right to expect that within its capacity a hospital must make reasonable response to the request of a patient for services. The hospital must provide evaluation, service, and/or referral indicated by the urgency of the case. When medically permissible the patient may be transferred to another facility only after he has received complete information and explanation concerning the needs for and alternatives to such a transfer. The institution to which the patient is to be transferred must first have accepted the patient for transfer.

continues

Table 5–1 *continued*

- The patient has the right to obtain information as to any relationship of his hospital to other health care and educational institutions insofar as his care is concerned. The patient has the right to obtain information as to the existence of any professional relationships among individuals, by name, who are treating him.

- The patient has the right to be advised if the hospital proposes to engage in or perform human experimentation affecting his care or treatment. The patient has the right to refuse to participate in such research projects.

- The patient has the right to expect reasonable continuity of care. He has the right to know in advance what appointment times and physicians are available and where. The patient has the right to expect that the hospital will provide a mechanism whereby he is informed by his physician or a delegate of the physician of the patient's continuing health care requirements following discharge.

- The patient has the right to examine and receive an explanation of his bill regardless of source of payment.

- The patient has the right to know what hospital rules and regulations apply to his conduct as a patient.

Reprinted with permission of the American Hospital Association.

VALUES AND ACCOUNTABILITY

A person's values influence beliefs about health, human needs, and illness, and human responses to illness. Nurses who work effectively with patients are sensitive to how a patient's values and their own values influence interactions. Values are formed over a lifetime from one's environment, culture, family, education, and profession.

A value is a belief about worth that acts as a standard to guide behavior. A value system is an organization of values where values are ranked along a continuum of importance. An attitude is a feeling or an emotion, usually including positive or negative judgment toward people, objects, and ideas. Beliefs are a class of attitudes primarily based on faith rather than fact. Both attitudes and beliefs influence human behavior and it is important to distinguish them from values.

There are several ways values are built and shared. These include moralizing, rewarding and punishing, modeling, laissez-faire, and responsible choice. Moralizing is the value system taught by parents or an institution that allows little opportunity for us to weigh different values. Rewarding and punishing are the positive and negative reinforcement that people receive for demonstrating positive values or when demonstrating inappropriate values. An example of rewarding and punishing is a parent scolding a child for pushing a sibling. Modeling represents how people absorb values by observing parents, significant others, and peers. Modeling can lead to socially acceptable or unacceptable behavior. Laissez-faire is an exploration of various values and the development of a personal value system. This may lead to problems and conflict because there is little or no guidance. Finally, through responsible choice people are encouraged to articulate different values and to examine the consequences involved.

Essential Nursing Values

The American Association of Colleges of Nursing has identified seven values (aesthetics, altruism, equality, freedom, human dignity, justice, and truth) and related attitudes and personal qualities.

Health care professionals are encouraged to respect and accept the individuality of patients. Nurses are encouraged to be "value neutral" and "nonjudgmental" in their various professional roles. The nurse does not assume that personal values are right and should not judge the patient's values as right or wrong depending on their congruence with the nurse's personal value system.

AN ETHICAL FRAMEWORK

Health care professionals must be able to use ethical thinking in their decision-making and clinical practice. Health care ethics pertain to how professionals fulfill their responsibilities and how care is provided to patients. Ethics are based on moral reasoning and reflects sets of values. Morals are standards of right and wrong that help individuals determine what is the appropriate or permissible action to take in a situation. Values are ideas or beliefs an individual considers important and feels strongly about. Values are developed through education, religious associations, family relationships, and friendship. Morals and values are the basis for establishing priorities and making choices.

Nurses must distinguish between personal values and professional ethics. Professional ethics involve principles that have universal application and standards of conduct that must be upheld in all situations. In ethical practice, a nurse avoids allowing personal judgment to bias treatment of patients. Professional ethics are the application of moral reasoning to all aspects of health care.

A Code for Nurses published by the American Nurses Association outlines the conduct and responsibilities nurses are expected to maintain in their practice. Ethical obligations include acting in the best interest of the patient, not only as individual practitioners, but also as members of the nursing profession, the health care team, and the community. A nurse is responsible to know and comply with the standards of ethical practice. The Code for Nurses is included in this chapter.

The foundations for ethical practice include knowledge of basic ethical concepts and the ability to understand their significance for professional responsibilities and patient care. Nurses committed to high-quality care base their practice on professional standards of ethical conduct. The study of professional ethical conduct begins in nursing school. It continues in discussions with colleagues and peers, and finally culminates when nurses pattern and absorb the behaviors of mentors who practice consistently with high ethical standards.

Nurses should understand the ethical theories that dictate and justify professional conduct. They also need to be familiar with codes of ethics, standards of practice, Patient Bill of Rights, and be skilled in using a model of ethical decision making to resolve ethical problems. Theory frameworks in ethics provide a systematic way of organizing reasons that are a basis for choosing the best actions. These theories may be broadly categorized as action-guiding theories that answer the question, "What should I do?" or character-guiding theories that answer the question, "What kind of person should I be?" Action-guiding theories fall into two main categories: (1) deontologic, an action is right or wrong independent of the outcomes it produces; (2) utilitarian, the correctness or wrongness of an action depends on the outcomes the action produces.

Major theoretical frameworks in ethics are differentiated according to the values emphasized as most important. Goals, duties, and rights are central considerations of all ethics theories, but they vary in how they are assigned priority within each of the frameworks.

In frameworks that emphasize goals, actions are judged to be right based on whether they contribute to the achievement of identified outcomes. In the utilitarian framework, actions are right when they contribute to the greatest good and wrong when they detract from the greatest good.

Some utilitarian theories define "good consequences" according to whether an action results in the greatest good for the greatest number. As an example, a decision could be made not to finance expensive experimental treatments needed by a few to reserve monies for wellness and prevention health programs and services that would benefit more people.

In the deontologic framework the emphasis is on a set of roles or responsibilities one is morally obligated to fulfill. One is expected to be committed to a specific set of duties, and these take priority over other considerations. Decisions about the correct action are based on which action is in keeping with these duties, not with regard to consequences. An example of a duty is the nurse's obligation to protect the privacy of the patient.

When rights are identified as the primary consideration, focus is on the claims or entitlements of each individual. Actions are judged according to whether they uphold each individual's rights. The advocacy of the "right to life" issue is an example of an ethical position based on rights.

Principles of Health Care Ethics

Principles are basic ideas that are a starting point for understanding and working through a problem. The major principles of health care ethics are beneficence, nonmaleficence, autonomy, and justice. These principles are the basis for rules that govern the relationships between health care professionals and patients.

Principle-Based Approach

The principle-based approach offers specific guidelines for practice.

Beauchamp and Childress' (1994) four-principles approach to ethics directs that we should act so as to respect the decision-making capacity of autonomous persons (**autonomy**); avoid causing harm (**nonmaleficence**); provide benefits and balance these benefits against risks and harms (**beneficence**); and distribute benefits, risks, and costs fairly (**justice**).

Autonomy means independence and the ability to be self-directed. In health care, respect for autonomy is the basis for the patient's right to self-determination, which means the patient is entitled to make decisions about what will happen to him or her and his or her body. Competent adult patients have the right to accept or refuse treatment. Even when the health care provider does not agree with the patient's decision, the patient's wishes must be respected. Nurses support patient autonomy by including the patient's wishes in the individualized treatment plan.

For patients who do not have the capacity for decision making about their health care, a surrogate decision-maker must be identified to act on behalf of the patient. **Advance directives** are documents that patients use to communicate their wishes to health care providers. These documents outline what treatment interventions the patient would or would not want if he or she became terminally ill, or if his or her ability to communicate or make decisions were impeded. A patient may designate another person to make decisions through the use of durable power of attorney for health care decisions (Figure 5–1). If the patient were unable to make decisions regarding health care, this decision-maker would act on the patient's behalf.

Patients are entitled to change their advance directives at any time. The nurse is obligated to document the patient's decision and to notify the other health care team members so that the patient's treatment may be modified to reflect the decision.

In attempting to support autonomy for the patient, health care providers must be sensitive to the implications of cultural diversity. The treatment plan must reflect respect for values or beliefs of various ethnic and social groups. Religious beliefs and traditions affect how much information a patient will share and how receptive he or she is to the treatment recommendations of the health care provider.

Nonmaleficence means to avoid doing harm. When working with patients, nurses must not cause injury or suffering. For example, nurses uphold the principle of nonmaleficence by preventing suffering by administering prescribed pain medications, or by preventing victimization from abuse through appropriate reporting mechanisms.

In some instances it is complex and difficult to discern issues surrounding helping the patient and avoiding harm. Saving the life of an expectant mother with a cardiac problem who is not likely to survive childbirth may require harm to the unborn child in the form of an abortion. Confronting a colleague who is a substance abuser may help the person obtain therapy and treatment; however, it may also mean a possible employment suspension and will likely cause embarrassment for the person.

Beneficence is working for and promoting good outcomes. Nurses and all health care practitioners work to accomplish good for patients by striving to achieve optimal patient outcomes. Nurses make beneficent actions when they administer pain medications, perform a dressing change, or provide emotional support to a patient who is anxious or depressed.

Justice, the principle of fairness, is the basis for the obligation to treat all patients in an equal and fair way. It is the foundation for decisions about resource allocation throughout a society or a group.

Nurses face issues of justice when organizing care for a group of patients and deciding how much time will be spent with each patient. A just decision is based on patient need and a fair distribution of resources. Nurses can identify ethical conflicts when a disruptive patient receives more attention than more cooperative ones. Another example of a justice issue is when a terminally ill patient receives life-sustaining treatment in a critical care unit, while another patient with a greater chance for recovery, cannot be admitted owing to lack of bed space. In these types of situations, nurses can promote justice by working with other members of the health care team in identifying realistic outcomes and developing a clearly defined treatment plan.

Issues of justice, such as how health care is funded, and whether all individuals have access to health care have implications for the community. Public policy must reflect just distribution of services. Nurses contribute their knowledge about patient care needs and the health care system to have an impact on serious decisions.

The principles of health care ethics must be upheld in all situations. They are the foundation for the ethical rules—veracity, fidelity, and confidentiality. These rules are the guidelines for the relationship between patients and health care providers (Figure 5–2).

Part I. Durable Power of Attorney for Health Care

- If you do NOT wish to name an agent to make health care decisions for you, write your initials in the box [Initials]

This form has been prepared to comply with the "Durable Power of Attorney for Health Care Act" of Missouri.

1. Selection of agent. I appoint:

Name: _____

Address: _____

[It is suggested that only one Agent be named. However, if more than one Agent is named, anyone may act individually unless you specify otherwise.]

Telephone: _____

as my Agent.

2. Alternate Agents. Only an Agent named by me may act under this Durable Power of Attorney. If my Agent resigns or is not able or available to make health care decisions for me, or if an Agent named by me is divorced from me or is my spouse and legally separated from me, I appoint the person(s) named below (in the order named if more than one):

First Alternate Agent   Second Alternate Agent

Name: _____   Name: _____

Address: _____   Address: _____

Telephone: _____   Telephone: _____

[This is a Durable Power of Attorney, and the authority of my Agent shall not terminate if I become disabled or incapacitated.]

Part I. Durable Power of Attorney for Health Care (Continued)

3. Effective date and durability. This Durable Power of Attorney is effective when two physicians decide and certify that I am incapacitated and unable to make and communicate a health care decision.

- If you want ONE physician, instead of TWO, to decide whether you are incapacitated, write your initials in the box to the right. [Initials]

4. Agent's powers. I grant to my Agent full authority to:

A. Give consent to, prohibit, or withdraw any type of health care, medical care, treatment, or procedure, even if my death may result;

- If you wish to AUTHORIZE your Agent to direct a health care provider to withhold or withdraw artificially supplied nutrition and hydration (including tube feeding of food and water), write your initials in the box to the right. [Initials]

- If you DO NOT WISH TO AUTHORIZE your Agent to direct a health care provider to withhold or withdraw artificially supplied nutrition and hydration (including tube feeding of food and water), write your initials in the box to the right. [Initials]

B. Make all necessary arrangements for health care services on my behalf, and to hire and fire medical personnel responsible for my care;

C. Move me into or out of any health care facility (even if against medical advice) to obtain compliance with the decisions of my Agent; and

D. Take any other action necessary to do what I authorize here, including (but not limited to) granting any waiver or release from liability required by any health care provider, and taking any legal action at the expense of my estate to enforce this Durable Power of Attorney.

5. Agent's Financial Liability and Compensation. My Agent acting under this Durable Power of Attorney will incur no personal financial liability. My Agent shall not be entitled to compensation for services performed under this Durable Power of Attorney, but my Agent shall be entitled to reimbursement for all reasonable expenses incurred as a result of carrying out any provision hereof.

Part II. Health Care Directive

• If you DO NOT WISH to make a health care directive, write your initials in the box to the right, and go to Part III. [Initials]

I make this HEALTH CARE DIRECTIVE ("Directive") to exercise my right to determine the course of my health care and to provide clear and convincing proof of my wishes and instructions about my treatment.

If I am persistently unconscious or there is no reasonable expectation of my recovery from a seriously incapacitating or terminal illness or condition, I direct that all of the life-prolonging procedures which I have initialed below be withheld or withdrawn.

I want the following life-prolonging procedures to be withheld or withdrawn:

• artificially supplied nutrition and hydration (including tube feeding of food and water). . . . . [Initials]

• surgery or other invasive procedures. . . . . [Initials]
• heart-lung resuscitation (CPR). . . . . [Initials]
• antibiotic. . . . . [Initials]
• dialysis. . . . . [Initials]
• mechanical ventilator (respirator). . . . . [Initials]
• chemotherapy. . . . . [Initials]
• radiation therapy. . . . . [Initials]
• all other "life-prolonging" medical or surgical procedures that are merely intended to keep me alive without reasonable hope of improving my condition or curing my illness or injury . . . . . [Initials]

However, if my physician believes that any life-prolonging procedure may lead to significant recovery, I direct my physician to try the treatment for a reasonable period of time. If it does not improve my condition, I direct the treatment be withdrawn even if it shortens my life. I also direct that I be given medical treatment to relieve pain or to provide comfort, even if such treatment might shorten my life, suppress my appetite or my breathing, or be habit forming.

IF I HAVE NOT DESIGNATED AN AGENT IN THE DURABLE POWER OF ATTORNEY, THIS DOCUMENT IS MEANT TO BE IN FULL FORCE AND EFFECT AS MY HEALTH CARE DIRECTIVE.

Part III. General Provisions Included in the Directive and Durable Power of Attorney

YOU MUST SIGN THIS DOCUMENT IN THE PRESENCE OF TWO WITNESSES.
IN WITNESS WHEREOF, I have executed this document this _____ day of _____, year _____.

_____
Signature

Print name _____
Address _____

The person who signed this document is of sound mind and voluntarily signed this document in our presence. Each of the undersigned witnesses is at least eighteen years of age.

Signature _____   Signature _____
Print name _____   Print name _____
Address _____   Address _____

ONLY REQUIRED FOR PART I — DURABLE POWER OF ATTORNEY

STATE OF MISSOURI)
) as
OF _____)

On this _____ day of _____, year _____, before me personally appeared to me known to be the person described in and who executed the foregoing instrument and acknowledged that he/she executed the same as his/her free act and deed.

IN WITNESS WHEREOF, I have hereunto set my hand and affixed my official seal in the County of _____, State of Missouri, the day and year first above written.

_____
Notary Public

My Commision Expires: _____

FIGURE 5–1 Durable power of attorney for health care and health care directive. *(Developed and printed by the Missouri Bar)*

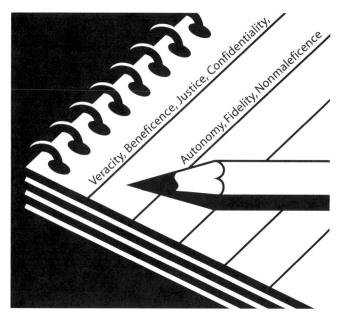

FIGURE 5-2 Principles of ethics

Veracity means upholding the truth and is essential to the patient-provider relationship. The right to self-determination is meaningless if the patient does not receive accurate, unbiased, and understandable information. Nurses help patients obtain information by arranging participation among the patient, the family, and the physician, and by providing emotional support to patients who are adjusting to illness. Patients would prefer accurate information about their condition and prognosis, even if the prognosis is bleak. Cancer patient studies show a large percentage of patients who want more information than what their physicians are inclined to reveal. These studies also show that informed patients are less anxious and more cooperative.

Fidelity means being faithful to one's commitments and promises. Nurses' commitments to patients include providing safe care and maintaining competence in nursing practice. Nurses must use discerning judgment when making promises to patients. It is important to be responsive to a patient's request, and the nurse must determine whether agreements can be upheld.

Confidentiality is the rule that requires patient information to be kept private. The patient's medical record is accessible only to those members of the health care team providing care to that patient. For patient information to be released, *a consent for release of information*

ASK YOURSELF

Veracity vs. Fidelity
It is important to be truthful while remaining faithful to the nurse-patient relationship. How do you respond to the patient who confides information to you, and you determine that it is important that the physician be aware of this information? What are the implications if you release the information to the physician? Is this a legal or ethical issue?

must be signed by the patient. The release must identify the person(s) to whom information is being released and for what purpose.

Breaking confidentiality may be ethically justified if there is a well-defined reason to share the information. Information may be shared only if this would substantially benefit someone else and if the benefit outweighs or overrides the harm that would come from a breach of confidentiality.

Ethical dilemmas arise when commitment to these principles suggests two conflicting courses of action. There is no foolproof method for identifying which principle is most important when there is conflict among competing principles.

Care-Based Approach

The nurse-patient relationship is primary to the care-based approach, which focuses attention to the "particulars" of individual patients who are viewed within the context of their lifestyle. The care perspective dictates that how the nurse chooses to be each time there is an encounter with a patient or a colleague is a matter of ethical significance. Characteristics of the care-based approach include: the caring relationship; respect the dignity and the patients as people; responding to others and to professional responsibility; defining moral skills to attentiveness, empathy, compassion; and respect of human individuality.

ADVOCACY

Advocacy is the protection and support of another's rights. For nurses, advocacy is a moral obligation and it is justified in both the principle- and care-based approaches to nursing ethics. Nurses who include advocacy as a part of their practice give priority to the good of the individual patient. They ensure that their loyalty to their employer or a colleague does not compromise their commitment to the patient. Finally, they evaluate autonomy and patient well-being.

When respecting patient well-being, the nurse acts in the best interest of the patient. When supporting autonomy, the nurse respects and supports the patient's right to make decisions. Both autonomy and patient well-being are promoted by each nurse in his or her nurse-patient relationships; however, it is possible for conflicts to arise. Nurses who are sensitive to the need to support and promote both autonomy and patient well-being are more likely to succeed in securing the patient's best interests.

RESOLVING DILEMMAS

Responsible ethical nursing practice includes managing oneself as a moral being, being an accountable employee in an organization, performing as a member of a health care team, and effectively participating in the community. In these areas, nurses must be able to recognize an ethical dilemma and then take the appropriate steps to resolve the issue. A dilemma exists when there are two or more choices available, the needs of the persons involved cannot be solved by the available options, and it is difficult to determine the best choice.

Ethical dilemmas in health care include issues regarding professional actions and patient care decisions. This can lead to conflict among members of the health care team. There are strategies nurses can use to prevent and resolve ethical dilemmas.

Case Considerations

When patients enter treatment, decisions must be made as to the most appropriate actions to take. Ethical issues are influential in all cases. Nurses must have the ability to analyze clinical situations to integrate ethical considerations with clinical data and surrounding issues. In making ethical decisions, health care professionals include several essential considerations. These assist in organizing the salient features of a clinical issue and facilitate problem solving and decision making. Case information may be divided into four categories: Indications for Medical Intervention, Patient Preference, Quality of Life, and Contextual Features (Table 5–2).

TABLE 5–2

Considerations for Case Analysis

Indications for Medical Intervention
- Patient's condition and prognosis
- Risks and benefits of intervention

What "good" can be done for the patient?

Patient Preference
- Consent or refusal of treatment
- Informed and competent

What are the patient's wishes?

Quality of Life
- Satisfaction with current situation
- Evaluation of future possibilities

Is it satisfying? Can it be improved?

Contextual Features
- Benefits and burdens for others
- Costs, policies, values of others

Is this use of resources justifiable?

Indications for Intervention

Indications for medical treatment include consideration of the patient's diagnosis and condition. Treatment options are evaluated based on whether they are indicated and what they may accomplish for the patient. The distinction between available treatment and the treatment that is truly indicated is important. The distinction must be based on whether the treatment option can achieve a therapeutic benefit for the patient. Beneficence and nonmaleficence are important considerations in this area. Judgment must be exercised about whether treatment will produce a benefit and what will achieve the best care for the patient. Nurses participate in this decision making by continually assessing the patient's condition and response to treatment and integrating this information into the plan of care. Available treatment interventions are not always beneficial for every patient.

Futility and Double Effect. Treatment interventions that probably will not preserve life, relieve suffering, or restore health are considered futile. Futility is usually defined in reference to the goals of the treatment plan; therefore, a treatment plan is designed based on the outcomes that are mutually agreed on by the patient and the health care practitioner.

Double effect means that an action may produce two outcomes. The outcome can be harmful and helpful at the same time. The reason for taking the action must be important enough to justify the negative consequences. For example, giving large doses of morphine to someone who is terminally ill may relieve the pain but it may also diminish respirations and hasten death. For example,

> A terminally ill patient with rectal bleeding, who has been told that he has approximately six months to live, is admitted through the emergency department to a medical-surgical unit. The primary care nurse has cared for this patient on previous admissions and is knowledgeable about the do-not-resuscitate orders for this patient. The physician on call has ordered blood replacement products as a part of the treatment plan of care. The nurse is concerned that resuscitation as a part of the treatment plan may be inappropriate, and that the goals of treatment need to be reviewed and discussed.

Patient Preference

The patient's input regarding medical care is essential to health care decision making. After clinical evaluation is completed and the clinical interventions have been determined, this information is given to the patient, who has the right to accept or refuse treatment alternatives. This is an expression of patient autonomy, and the wishes of an informed, competent patient must always be included in the individualized patient treatment plan.

> In the patient care case example discussed earlier, if the physician planned to administer the blood products and the patient did not want the treatment and had discussed this with the nurse, the nurse should advocate for the patient's wishes and inform the physician. Even though the physician believes that treatment would provide therapeutic gain for the patient, the patient's preference must be respected.

Informed Consent. Patients have a right to make decisions about the care they will receive. To make appropriate decisions, the patient must have information about his or her condition, the suggested treatment, the various risks and benefits associated with the treatment, and any alternative treatment modalities. Informed and valid consent is a process of shared decision making with respect and participation.

As a patient advocate, the nurse must listen carefully to the patient to determine if the patient needs additional information or clarification. Ethical nursing practice is to advocate for the patient by answering questions or accommodating the patient's need for time to adjust to the information provided. These nursing actions will help to ensure that the patients' wishes are known and included in the decisions regarding the treatment plan.

Quality of Life

Quality of life refers to how satisfying a person's life is according to his or her point of view. The patient evaluates his or her experience and determines the quality according to his or her own personal standards. Some patients feel that life is not worth living if they cannot return to their preferred activities, whereas others make adjustments and live within their adapting limits.

Nurses assess a patient's quality of life when they observe how a patient is managing or adapting to the constraints of an illness or injury. Nurses need to make clinical judgments about the quality of life in light of the required adjustment. Some patients prefer to be independent and will, therefore, experience a greater sense of loss and may be less satisfied with the quality of life than someone who readily accepts assistance and has a support system available.

Contextual Features

Benefits or burdens that affect individuals or groups other than the patient but have compelling influence on a situation are called contextual features. Factors included are finances, availability and use of resources, family situations, influence of family or friends, and organizational or public policy.

The influence of these factors may be demonstrated by reviewing a patient's case from differing perspectives. A child born with several congenital anomalies will require extensive surgeries to survive, with lengthy, numerous hospitalizations requiring intensive care. This child may benefit from a stable family environment, a secure family income,

ASK YOURSELF

When providing care to your patients, what impact does their lifestyle have on the way you provide care? For example, what if the patient has a sexually transmitted disease, or is an unmarried teenage mother, or is homeless?

and health care insurance. On the other hand, this child might be born to a single mother who finds it difficult to look at the child and wants to relinquish her parental rights to a state child care agency.

The case involves a dilemma about whether to provide life-sustaining treatment for a child with severe health problems. The decision to treat this child becomes more complex because of the problems that will remain after extensive treatment interventions. The contextual features would be considered in deciding on the best course of action for the child.

Conduct a Case Analysis

In making difficult ethical decisions the case analysis model may be adopted. It organizes the facts of a case and clarifies the ethical issues that should be considered. Case analysis may be completed by members of the health care team or the organization's ethics committee may provide assistance. Information about the case is shared through the team conference format.

Identify Outcomes

The patient's individualized treatment and care plan requires focus and consistency and planning is essential. Ethical conflicts may arise because of differences about the goals of the treatment plan. Realistic outcomes need to be established when all of the information is considered.

Analyze and Diagnose

In a specific ethical situation, the various individual health care team members have different roles and information to contribute to the case management and analysis. The nurse shares information about the patient's adaptation to illness and response to treatment. The physician contributes facts about the patient's medical condition and prognosis. Various therapists contribute information about how the patient's capabilities will affect the quality of life. Social services members provide information about community resources.

When all of the information about a case is gathered, problems and issues can be identified and clarified. Ethical conflicts can be identified, the significance of various factors is evident, and options can be viewed in light of the specifics of that case.

Identify Accountabilities

Different members of the health care team are accountable for actions that have been identified as part of the patient's treatment plan. For example, if there are questions about medical conditions and treatment response, the physician may need to pursue additional diagnostics or consultations. If the patient has a living will, the nurse may contact the social worker, who will contact the family and request a copy of the document. When the patient's preferences are unclear, a psychosocial specialist may be contacted to work with the patient to determine what he or she wants or hopes for from the medical treatment.

Identify Goals

The treatment outcomes for a patient with a terminal illness may include such goals as pain relief, advance directives regarding a surrogate decision-maker, resuscitation efforts, and hospice care. Clarifying actions to be taken in relation to each of these concerns promotes a sense of well-being for the patient. Answers to these questions can prevent confusion about the care to be provided, and health care team members can prevent crisis management. An effective treatment results from realistic and desirable goals rather than allowing the situation to become more complex without a viable plan.

Follow Through

When a plan is established and there is agreement by the patient, health care professionals are ethically bound to uphold their accountabilities and responsibilities by following through with their part of the plan. Failing to follow through undermines the public's trust in health care professionals.

Health care decisions can involve a significant number of considerations and they can be complex. The complexities involved can add to the emotional reactions of those involved. By working through feelings to an event and discussing feelings and reactions among the team members, health care professionals can learn from the experience. This kind of discussion can help in planning care for future patients and preventing residual feelings from deterring their ability to work through similar situations in the future.

ETHICS COMMITTEES

Many health care institutions have organizational ethics committees whose primary functions include policy making, case review, education, and consultation. The American Hospital Association encourages the development of these committees as interdisciplinary vehicles for identifying and addressing ethical issues. These committees are specifically equipped to deal with the complexities and challenges of health care because they are interdisciplinary and provide a vehicle where different views may be aired without fear of repercussion.

Nurses bring an essential voice to the ethics committee. When cases are being discussed, nurses help to ensure that the technical facts are understood, the appropriate decision-makers are identified, the patient's medical best interests are identified, and the course of action selected is justified by sound ethical principles (Figure 5–3).

Nurses also play an important role in policy making. They are frequently able to identify what policies are needed to address current ethical concerns and to suggest needed modifications of existing policies.

SPECIFIC ETHICAL ISSUES

Staffing shortages often mean too few nurses for the number and acuity of patients in a unit. Understaffing may also mean unlicensed assistive personnel in questionable assignments, or it may mean nurses assigned to a unit are not familiar with the patients and procedures. This is a very dangerous trend.

Short-staffing carries inherent risks, and nurses may be held accountable for mistakes related to understaffing. Nurses must take action to protect the patients and the staff. Several safeguards are discussed in Table 5–3.

Mechanical Life Support

Medical technological advancement frequently allows patients to be systematically maintained for sustained periods of time. The contro-

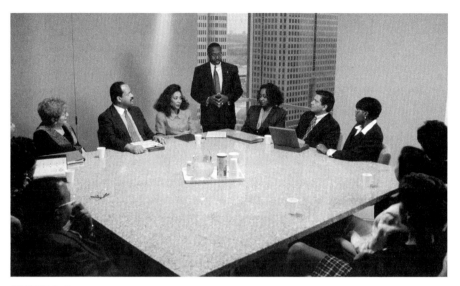

FIGURE 5-3 Ethics committee meeting *(Photo courtesy of Photodisc)*

versial question is, should death be delayed? Another question is, what is death? The answers can vary from state to state, and a traditional definition of death (both pulse and respiration absent) has become debatable.

Patients who sign advance directives and living wills provide directions regarding life-sustaining issues. The presence or absence of an

---

TABLE 5-3

Surviving Staffing Shortages

- Be sure to inform the nurse-manager, including the number of staff and patients in the unit, and the patients' acuity levels.
- Properly prioritize the needs of patients in your care, making sure that seriously ill patients receive priority.
- Know your hospital's policy on floating. If you are assigned to a unit where you feel you are not prepared to provide safe care, discuss the assignment with your nurse-manager.
- Assist a nurse who has been assigned to your unit by offering to work as a team.
- Do not leave the unit if you become frustrated. You could be charged with abandoning your patients.

---

advance directive or a living will must be documented in the patient's record. When caring for patients on life support, the nurse must be aware of state laws regarding the definition of death and the legally binding nature of living wills. Nurses should document any statements regarding a patient's convictions, intentions, and continued desire to refuse treatment.

Organ Transplantation

The Uniform Anatomical Gift Act allows the patient to sign a donor card, willing some or all of his or her organs after death. The number of transplants is increasing because of improvements in tissue typing, improved surgical techniques, and increased success with immuno-logic suppressant pharmaceuticals.

When organ transplant is a viable option, the well-being and quality of life of both the donor and the recipient must be considered. Factors influencing the decision include one's social, cultural, and religious beliefs and values.

Although there is an increasing public awareness of successful organ transplants, body mutilation before or after death is an expressed concern. Other ethical questions raised include: How are the resources assigned and who decides? How are the financial resources allocated? The nurse's role in this issue includes answering questions and referring patients and families to appropriate members of the health care team for resolution of issues. Providing objective information and all available resources to patients and families is an essential responsibility of the nurse.

Health Care Rationing

In the United States, many people are uninsured or underinsured, or have limited access to health care. A continued subject of debate is whether each person has a "right" to basic health care. To complicate matters, given the rapid advancement of medical technology, there is now even a debate among health care professionals regarding what constitutes "basic" coverage. Rationing health care could limit options available to the elderly, the terminally ill, the poor, and to those in society many view as having limited "social value." How can nurses ensure that their voices and the nursing viewpoint are heard?

Nurse Incompetence

Reporting a colleague is never easy; however, it is a responsibility to patients and a commitment to nursing ethics and conduct. When considering a situation, it must be carefully evaluated. Questions to consider may include: Has the conduct harmed the patient? Is the action the result of incompetence or ethical in nature? It is difficult at best to answer these questions, and nurses must consider the consequences of any actions taken. These guidelines may be helpful:

- Always follow proper channels.
- Be specific, clear, and factual in documentation.
- Be open and consistent.
- Document all actions taken.
- Continue to follow proper channels and procedures.

Before taking any action, it is advisable to discuss the situation with the nurse directly. Share the concern about the possible consequences of his or her conduct. If the outcome of your discussion is not satisfactory, then consult a trusted professional, the nurse manager, or a member of the ethics committee and follow an appropriate course of action.

Chemical Abuse

A Nursing Task Force on Addiction and Psychological Disturbance was appointed by the American Nurses Association in the early 1980s. The purpose of the task force was to develop guidelines for treatment and assistance for nurses whose alcoholism, drug abuse, or psychological problems interfere with their nursing practice. The guidelines were developed for use by state nurses' associations.

What are some of the behaviors or symptoms exhibited by the chemically impaired nurse? They may include:

- an increase in charting errors
- personality changes, mood swings
- changes in behavior and mental status
- inappropriate charting
- increased absenteeism and inability to meet scheduled work shifts
- complaints of poor pain control from assigned patients
- unsteady gait, flushed face
- alcohol on the breath, slurred speech

Fortunately, nursing has become increasingly sensitive to the issues surrounding the chemically abusive nurse, and through professional associations, efforts are now devoted to providing the assistance necessary.

What is the proper course of behavior regarding a nurse suspected of abuse? Nursing professionals suggest that the colleague not be confronted. Gather information and make certain that a problem does exist. Follow your agency's policies and procedures in the matter. Many health care organizations have ethics committees that can be consulted for assistance.

Investigation of the situation will continue, and if a problem does exist, appropriate actions will be taken. Some states have referral systems in place for nurses with treatment plans and rehabilitation programs. When chemical abuse is suspected, ignoring it or protecting a colleague is the worst "favor" the nurse can give. Consider the ramifications of job loss, malpractice lawsuits, harm to patients, and disciplinary action by the licensing agency.

Reporting a colleague is a difficult and complex situation. There may be personal and professional implications. Nurses must remember that the integrity of nursing and public trust must be maintained. There are several qualities of a profession and one of the most significant is its ability to safeguard its standards of quality through self-monitoring.

KEY POINTS

- Nurses must use ethical reasoning in their nursing practice.
- Ethical dilemmas involve choosing between conflicting values, resolving a dilemma-structured analysis based on moral principles.
- A value is a belief about worth that acts as a standard to guide behavior.
- Values are formed over a lifetime from information a person receives from the environment, the family, and culture. Common modes of transmission are moralizing, modeling, laissez-faire, rewarding and punishing, and responsible choice.
- Values influence beliefs about human needs, health and illness, the practice of health-related behaviors, and human responses to health and illness.
- Essential values for the practicing nurse include aesthetics, equality, freedom, altruism, human dignity, justice, and truth.
- Ethics offers the nurse a means to look at and evaluate alternative courses of right action, using basic moral concepts and principles.
- Ethics theories offer moral guides to action and to character. Nurse ethicists frequently use two theoretical and practical approaches to ethics, the principle-based approach and the care-based approach.
- Values clarification is a process by which people come to understand their own values and value systems.

▦ Nursing codes of ethics provide a framework for making ethical decisions and set forth professional expectations. They inform both the nurse and society of the profession's primary goals and values. Codes are effective only when upheld by members of the profession.

▦ Nurses can serve on institutional ethics committees whose primary functions include policy formulation, education, consultation, and case review.

CRITICAL THINKING ACTIVITIES

1. A mother delivers a baby with several congenital problems. The baby's prognosis is poor and he is not expected to live more than a few months. During the team conference, the parents state that they cannot afford to pay for the infant's care. How is the degree of intervention determined? Who makes the decision? What factors are the basis for the decision?

2. The principle of autonomy refers to the individual's right to choose and the ability to act on that choice. Patients have a right to self-determination, even when their decisions result in self-harm. Discuss how you as a nurse will support the patient's right to refuse treatment.

   Discuss the principle of autonomy and how you feel about the following patient behaviors:

   continuing to drink alcohol with a diagnosis of cirrhosis
   refusing to take medications
   smoking with a diagnosis of lung cancer or emphysema

➡ CASE STUDY

Lee Stokes, a nurse with several years' nursing experience, has been working part-time for three weeks in a small rural hospital. She is the evening charge nurse on the pediatric floor for two evenings a week and on a surgical floor the third evening. On a busy shift one evening, a patient on the surgical unit was supposed to receive phenobarbital gr.¼. Lee mistakenly administered codeine gr.¼ to the patient. At the end of the shift, Lee counted narcotics with the oncoming shift nurse, Kathy. As Kathy

continues

CASE STUDY *continued*

counted aloud the remaining narcotics and barbiturates, Lee wrote the same total that had previously been noted for each, rather than writing the actual count. She did not realize what she had done.

The next night, Kathy brought the matter of the extra phenobarbital and the missing codeine to Lee's attention, told Lee that she had "goofed," and said that she had fixed Lee's error during the night. She had "jimmied" the books by throwing away a phenobarbital and by falsely writing in the codeine book that she had given codeine gr. ¼ to a patient who conveniently had an order for it.

Lee does not know if she should report her mistake. On the one hand, she thinks she can overlook her medication error because the patient was not harmed and, although Kathy knows of the mistake, it is doubtful that others will discover it. By not reporting her error to the nursing administration, Lee could keep her total number of incident reports low. She knows that many nurses in the hospital believe that other nurses interpret a low number of incident reports as "no error" nursing, which, they believe, is synonymous with "good" nursing. On the other hand, Lee knows that as an honest person she should report her error, and she believes that honesty is an important part of her professional identity. Further, she believes that she should follow hospital policy and rules. But in admitting her mistake, she would expose Kathy's cover-up activities, including the falsification of narcotic records.

Among the questions raised in this case are:

To what extent, if any, should a nurse jeopardize his/her own or another's professional position by admitting an error?

Must a nurse report a cover-up in order to maintain one's authority as a nurse and effectiveness as a role model?

Some basic information about relationships among nurses is necessary for a discussion of this case. Various general factors affect relationships between nurses. These include remnants of the historical legacy of nursing, technological and social changes, the expanding scope of nursing practice, the ideology of professionalism, and the increased importance of education.

BIBLIOGRAPHY

American Hospital Association. (1992). *A Patient's Bill of Rights.* Chicago: Author.

American Nurses Association. (1985). *Code for nurse with interpretive statements.* Kansas City, MO: Author.

Awong, L., & Miles, A. (1998a). When the physician disregards the patient's expressed wishes. *American Journal of Nursing, 98*(2), 71.

Benjamin, M., & Curtis, J. (1986). *Ethics in nursing.* New York: Oxford University Press.

Creighton, H. (1986). *Law every nurse should know* (5th ed.). Philadelphia: W. B. Saunders.

Haddad, A. (1995). Ethics in action. *RN, 58*(5), 21–23.

Haddad, A. (1998). Ethics in action. *RN, 61*(3), 21–24.

Jonsen, A. R., Siegler, M., & Winslade, W. (1992). *Clinical ethics* (3rd ed.). New York: McGraw-Hill.

Munson, R. (1992). *Intervention and reflection: Basic issues in medical ethics* (4th ed). Belmont, CA: Wadsworth.

President's Commission for the Study of Ethical Problems in Medicine and Biomedical Behavioral Research. (1982). Washington, DC: U.S. Government Printing Office.

Rice, V. H., Bech, C., & Stevenson, J. S. (1997). Ethical issues relative to autonomy and personal control in independent and cognitively impaired elders. *Nursing Outlook, 45*(1), 25–34.

Silva, M. C. (1990). Preparation of nurse executives for ethical decision making. *Nursing Connections, 3*(2), 28–31.

Singer, P. A., Pellegrino, E. D., & Siegler, M. (1990). Ethics committees and consultants. *Journal of Clinical Ethics, 1*(4), 263–267.

Zollo, M. B., & Derse, A. (1997). The abusive patient: Where do you draw the line? *American Journal of Nursing, 97*(2), 31–35.

INTERNET RESOURCES

Bioethics for Clinicians
    http://www.cma.ca/cmaj/series/bioethic.htm
Hospice Hands
    http://www.hospice-cares.com
Medweb
    http://www.medweb.emory.edu/medweb

CHAPTER 6

Critical Thinking in Nursing Practice

⟹ **OVERVIEW**

Critical thinking is a vital aspect of nursing. The nursing process is in many ways critical thinking applied. However, because it is often defined in many ways, clarification of this concept is important. Discussion in this chapter includes the influences on thought, the stumbling blocks to judgment, and the critical factors influencing thinking. The factors affecting the "doing" of nursing will be paralleled with the nursing process.

⟹ **OBJECTIVES**

Upon completion of this chapter, the reader should be able to:

■ Assess the impact of thinking on learning and the practice of nursing.
■ Classify the ways of thinking.
■ Discuss how thinking and doing are intertwined.
■ Examine the factors that affect doing.
■ Define the components of the nursing process and the thinking and doing related to each component.

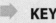

KEY TERMS

Content knowledge	NANDA
Habits	Patient
Inquiry	

INTRODUCTION

Clinical judgment and critical thinking are essential for nurses. When married to the nursing process, they enable the use of intellectual, interpersonal, and technical skills to succeed in nursing. Critical thinking is sometimes defined as an inquiry, which is a questioning approach to issues. This is too narrow. Critical thinking is active and dynamic. It involves a constant reappraisal and reanalysis of a situation because as conditions change so might the best solution. A smart nurse is always monitoring his or her activities. The result is always the same: better outcomes for patients and practitioners.

THINKING AND THE WAYS OF THINKING

All people are not the same. It stands to reason that the way they process information should differ as well. The way they think about the information is different too. It is clear that it is not easy to categorize the thought process into a neat package or box.

Thinking is not a static process; it changes daily, even hourly. Because it is so dynamic (constantly changing) and there are no nursing actions that do not require a high degree of thought and analysis, it is important to understand thinking in general. It is also important to assess one's own unique styles and patterns and to identify strategies for effective critical thought.

In the process of making frequent large and small decisions throughout the day, people will occasionally think of options and alternatives. For the most part, however, people make many (if not most) decisions without giving much thought to the issue. Yet, each of the options or alternatives may provide a better result. Unfortunately, all too often people rely on past habits or approaches to solve a problem. Staying mentally alert and open to new circumstances allow nurses to think of and honestly consider changes.

INFLUENCES ON THOUGHT

The influences on thought can be divided into four broad areas. These are: (1) intelligence, (2) memory, (3) environmental conditions, and (4) personality.

Intelligence

Intellectual ability determines a person's understanding of problems and the methods individuals use to solve them. This ability also determines the speed and accuracy of our performance.

Memory

Memory is a shorthand for information stored from past experiences. It helps individuals recognize and produce what is required in a particular situation. The circumstances of those experiences frequently influence the selection and organization of responses.

Environmental Conditions

A given task, and the demands it makes, strongly determine the efficiency of a person's performance. For example, a nurse influenced by the difficulty and complexity of a situation may be under a high degree of stress and not working efficiently.

Personality

Certain internal factors also influence thought and problem solving. They include an individual's emotional state, motivation, and attitudes. These conditions determine how strongly aroused one must be to perform well, and the degree to which the task causes anxiety or worry. These factors also determine how effectively a person can control or direct his or her response in relation to the situation.

CLASSIFYING THINKING MODES

Many people have tried to explain the thought process and thinking by developing classification systems. One example is "The Six Rs"—remembering, repeating, reasoning, reorganizing, relating, and reflecting. Although the six Rs are a useful tool, thinking styles used in nursing are better represented by a somewhat different classification system. The five modes are total recall, habits, inquiry, new ideas and creativity, and self-awareness (Figure 6–1).

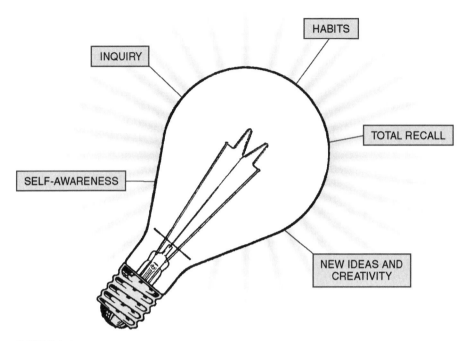

FIGURE 6-1 Modes of thinking

The best thinkers—and the best nurses—use all of these modes at one time. This may seem impossible, but it is important to note that these modes are not used individually so much as in combination with each other. Every student nurse discovers at one time or another that nursing has few aspects that fit into clearly delineated, mutually exclusive categories; however, before a unified way of thinking may be understood, each aspect should be examined individually, keeping in mind that each one is rarely used alone.

Total Recall

Total recall means remembering facts, such as the date the Crimean War ended, normal frequently used blood laboratory values, who Florence Nightingale was, and so on. These are important things. Nurses use total recall by either remembering the facts or recollecting where to look for them.

How total one's recall is depends on memory. Memory is a complex process. Some people can remember many seemingly isolated facts effortlessly; others struggle. There are many ways to help people who struggle with remembering. Putting facts into patterns is one way.

Mnemonics is one example (using a pattern to help recall a larger pattern of information). For instance, a common first aid mnemonic device is "RICE." This helps many people respond immediately to many first aid situations with "rest," "ice," "compression," and "elevation." Often, however, patterns are not quite so obvious. Individuals often have to make or find the patterns to use them. For example, at first glance the numbers "3238183264" are meaningless. However, when the same numbers are considered this way "(323) 818-3264," the picture becomes clear. It is a telephone number. The numbers are easier to remember because there is a familiar pattern to them.

The way people receive information also affects their ability to recognize patterns. A simple test is to make a list of items that may be readily categorized. The list should be mixed up and read to another individual. Can he or she remember them? Show the person the written words in the order that they were read and see if he or she can remember them now. Which way is easier? Could the person recognize the patterns more quickly when hearing or when seeing? This is a valuable test for everyone to take. Learning how one's mind processes information is a valuable bit of knowledge. The experience will provide a clue on how to study and learn the mountains of "facts" a nurse needs to remember as both a nursing student and as a graduate nurse.

Another process for remembering is the association of a fact with some experience. Most people who were at least ten years old at the time remember exactly what they were doing when President John Kennedy was shot. Other associations are less dramatic. A student may remember something heard in a lecture because the instructor supported the fact with a funny story.

Habits

Habits are accepted patterns of actions that experience has shown to be effective. They work. They effectively manage time, or are necessary. Habits are thinking approaches that are repeated so often they are second nature. The great advantage of habits is that they allow people to finish a task without having to figure out a new method each time. Riding a bicycle and driving a car are habits for most people (Figure 6–2). It is not uncommon for people to drive several miles and then realize they could not recall what they saw or what streets they passed. This "mindless" driving is possible because most adults have already mastered the basic mechanics of driving and can do it without conscious effort.

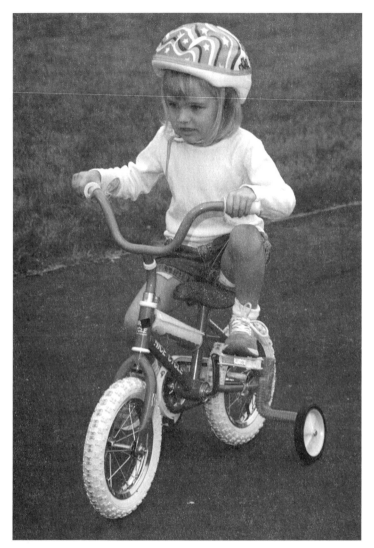

FIGURE 6–2 Riding a bike is a habit for most people. Nurses develop many useful habits that serve them well in practice.

Cardiopulmonary resuscitation (CPR) is a very useful habit in nursing. When someone is lying on the ground in obvious distress, there is no time to come up with a creative way to revive him or her. A quick solution is needed. Nursing has many other procedures comparable to CPR—the proper way to give an injection, take a temperature, insert a catheter, and many more such activities. When these actions are first learned, they obviously are not yet habits, but as they are used repeatedly, they become second nature: They become habits.

Inquiry

Inquiry is the process of examining issues in depth and questioning that which may seem immediately obvious. Inquiry is the primary kind of thinking used to reach conclusions. Conclusions can be reached without using inquiry, but conclusions are better (more accurate) if inquiry is used. For example, a student sitting at her desk looked at her window and saw that it was wet. Her immediate conclusion was, "It's raining and I won't be able to go to the beach when I'm done studying." On a closer look, she saw that there was no water on the grass; the sun was shining; there were no clouds; and there was a ladder visible on the side of the window. This struck her as odd so she looked at the window from a different angle. She thought that someone may have left a sprinkler on. From the new perspective she was relieved to see a window washer cleaning nearby windows. With all of the information, she came to the most accurate conclusion—the windows were being washed. In this example, inquiry was used when the student did the following:

- saw something (received information)
- came to an immediate conclusion
- collected additional information to rule in or rule out the first idea (immediate conclusion)
- compared new information to what was already known about a situation like this by using past experience
- questioned any biases
- considered one or more alternative conclusions
- validated the original or the alternative conclusion

This process of collecting and analyzing information to confirm or to make additional conclusions beyond the obvious ones is the essence of inquiry.

In the story provided, the example is fairly simple. In nursing, things are more complex. Most situations in nursing practice require inquiry. Sometimes a single validated conclusion emerges; at other times, several conclusions may seem equally valid. In those cases, a nurse needs to repeat the inquiry until the one conclusion that is most accurate is found. This sounds very time consuming, and in some cases it is, but in most situations the process occurs in microseconds, especially for experienced nurses. Many experts refer to this process as diagnostic reasoning. Consider this example of a nursing situation:

During the night shift in an acute care hospital, the nurse notices a patient's room light is on. She enters the room, speaks to the patient, and states, "I noticed your room light on, how are you doing?" The patient responds, "I'm doing fine." The nurse notices that there are tissues on the patient's bedside table and that the patient's eyes are red and puffy.

Inquiry is needed. The nurse must make a preliminary conclusion about something that is not readily apparent. The patient is smiling and saying nothing is wrong. Should the nurse accept the patient's response and conclude he is fine? Not if she was using inquiry. She would put several pieces of information together to make some sense out of the situation. The nurse would recognize that there may be no simple answer, but several possible conclusions. Using inquiry allows the nurse to consider at least the following four conclusions:

1. The patient is fine. He is normally awake at this hour, and may have been rubbing his eyes because of his allergies.
2. The patient is fine but can't sleep because he was bored and napped all day. His eyes are always red and puffy.
3. The patient is not fine but doesn't want to talk about it or bother anyone.
4. The patient is not fine but doesn't know how to ask for help.

To say with any degree of certainty that one of these four conclusions is better than the others, the nurse needs to validate her conclusion. She needs to put together as much information as possible, and to ask the patient directly if he agrees with the final conclusion. To get the necessary information, the nurse must ask questions and observe reactions and the surroundings. She needs to analyze the information by looking for patterns and determining what was significant. Determining significance is dependent on the nurse's ability to think about how the information about the patient compares to the nursing content knowledge she has learned.

Content knowledge or factual knowledge from textbooks (total recall) is not enough. Answers to many situations are not always found in a book. Books help nurses see patterns by providing factual information, such as usual behavior patterns or the appearance of the eyes, but each nurse has to put that material together with the information found in each unique situation. Books describe the usual ways to interpret information and the usual rules, but not everyone or every situation fits into these usual patterns (norms). For example, most people are asleep during the nighttime hours, but not all; most people's eyes are not red and puffy, but some people's eyes are. It is necessary to use inquiry to collect key information and put the pieces together in meaningful patterns. Books cannot do this.

New Ideas and Creativity

New ideas and creativity compose a thinking mode that is very special. This individualized thinking goes beyond the usual to reconfigure the norm. Like inquiry, this mode allows people to go beyond textbook ideas. True creative thinking is at the opposite end of the spectrum from the *Habit* mode. Instead of saying, "This is the way things have always been done," the creative thinker says, "Let's try this new way." Creative thinking is not for the faint-hearted; one must be willing to take risks and buck the established order. Many people are discouraged from being creative. Peer pressure is powerful. No one wants to be "different from the rest of the crowd"; however, everybody is creative under certain circumstances.

New ideas and creativity are very important in nursing because they are at the root of individualized care. Many things nurses learn have to be mixed, matched, and reworked to fit each unique patient situation. Nursing has many standard approaches to care that save time and generally work well, but they do not work the same way for everyone. For example, a female patient who resides in a long-term care facility spends her time wheeling herself up and down the hallways in her wheelchair. The nurses repeatedly give her verbal prompting and she does not respond. Most nurses think of therapeutic communication as talking to the patient and they respond as a participant in the communication process. One of the nurses decided to try something different and one day, she approached the patient, gave her a hug, smiled, and said, "Let's sing." The patient responded by singing. No one knew that she could sing.

Other nurses knew about the standards for therapeutic communication, and they used them with the best of intentions. Standard verbal approaches to therapeutic communication work well with most patients. The nurse, however, expanded the definition of therapeutic communication to include singing and touching, thus creating an individualized approach for this patient that was not included in the textbooks. One small, creative approach that individualizes care often has a way of mushrooming into bigger and better things.

Self-awareness

Self-awareness (or knowing how one thinks) is roughly defined as thinking about one's thinking. This is "metacognition," a word meaning (meta) "among or in the midst of," and (cognition), which means "the process of knowing."

Awareness of one's own thought process is somewhat difficult for most people because there are specific analytical terms used to describe how we think. Few people ever learn this specialized vocabulary. When assessing one's own thought process, it is necessary to investigate personal assumptions and preferences. What perspectives and biases do I, as an individual, possess?

Table 6–1 provides a list of the words used to describe how one thinks. A good exercise is to review this list and select the commonly used words. Pay particular attention to how these terms are used. Learning the language and using these thought processes is foreign to most people and it requires reaching a level of comfort with the new words and the thinking that is associated with it. The five modes of

TABLE 6–1

Glossary for Thinking About Thinking

Ambiguous (ambiguity): unclear, having multiple meanings

Assume (assumption): take for granted

Bias: a neutral, negative, or positive inclination

Conclude (conclusion): make a judgment or decision based on reasoning

Contradict (contradiction): state an opposing view, deny

Credible (credibility): worthy of belief or trust

Distinguish: recognize plainly by the senses; to separate and classify

Elaborate (elaboration): expand on

Evidence: data that support conclusion

Infer (inference): a strong or weak, justified or unjustified conclusion based on information and assumptions

Interpret (interpretation): explain the meaning of, make understandable

Justify (justification): to show to be just, right, or in accord with reason

Point of view: perspective; one's personal way of looking at the world based on background and experiences

Relevance: importance, significant relationship

Validate (validation): to verify, to search for evidence to support a conclusion

thinking need to be used together, and it is essential to discuss some of the "stumbling blocks" to unified thinking as well as factors that make each person's thinking unique.

STUMBLING BLOCKS TO THINKING

One of the most obvious stumbling blocks is *getting into a rut,* and the most common way of getting into a rut is to overuse the *habit* mode. At the beginning of their nursing program, student nurses do not have nursing habits, but these are quickly developed. Habits provide security and comfort, so they have a definite value. Nurses need habits. Beginning nurses follow recipes at first to provide safe, basic nursing care; otherwise they are unsafe.

Problems occur, however, when nurses stop *thinking* after they have developed some comfortable, secure, and safe habits of patient care. Habits do feel good but they also discourage the use of inquiry and new ideas. One needs to be a risk-taker to think beyond habits. Taking risks means being willing to question what is read and heard. Questioning expands one's awareness and solidifies new knowledge. One risk of questioning is that it may be interpreted as defiance. Defiance is focused on the power of the authority figure rather than on the information being provided by those sources. Focusing on the issues instead of the source of information decreases the risk of misinterpretation.

Nurses care for patients who do not fit the textbook recipe as closely as books say they will. When that happens, it is necessary to use other modes of thinking to find the alternative explanations and creative interventions. This is called individualization. As health care consumers, most people would not want the health care professional to approach them only with habits and recipes, and presume they are exactly like everybody else in the textbook.

Anxiety is another significant stumbling block to thinking. Increased anxiety shuts down and limits inquiry and new ideas and creativity. Those new to nursing practice often find it to be a frightening experience that provokes anxiety. The pressure of adjusting and adapting to new procedures, new language, new ways of writing, new books, and unstable schedules can be unsettling. Anxiety decreases one's thinking abilities, even about simple things like talking. Imagine what anxiety can do to critical thinking challenges such as problem solving and learning. Learning and problem solving compose 90 percent of nurse thinking, so it is worthwhile to find ways to decrease anxiety.

FACTORS INFLUENCING THINKING

Everyone is unique and brings feelings, backgrounds, ideas, values, and cultures to his or her thinking. Some of the key factors influencing thinking are discussed here.

Consistency

In the ideal world, nurses would switch on their critical thinking skills, turn up the power to high, and always (consistently) be great thinkers. In the real world, however, many things interfere with this rosy picture. Food, beverage, room temperature, lighting, clothing, energy levels, sleep deprivation, illness, and many other factors create peaks and valleys. Sometimes thinkers are "sharp as a tack"; other times they are "dense as fog." It is important for nurses to recognize the inconsistencies in their thinking and be aware of what helps and what hinders them to maximize their best thinking times.

Organization

What is perceived as organized by one person may seem disorganized to another. The important thing is for each individual to find the organizational patterns that work best for himself or herself. Some people need lists; others need various notes pasted in strategic places of high visibility; whereas others will mentally store items. Each person needs to identify the style that works best for him or her and then work to improve it.

Memory

The discussion on total recall earlier in this chapter may be reviewed for information on memory. Remembering isolated facts, new idea association with things already known, peak experiences needed to aid in remembering, and memory aids, are all considerations when it is recalled how people remember things and for how long.

Feelings

Feelings, or emotions, are usually identified in one word: mad, sad, glad, happy, frustrated, confused, angry, elated, scared, anxious, and so on. Feelings are a part of life; they cannot and should not be ignored. But one can learn to recognize them. The effect that emotions have on one's thinking can be recognized. It is important to develop ways to modify the circumstances that contribute to the feelings.

Intuition

This is a "gut feeling." Historically, the nursing profession has discouraged the use of intuition, stating that it was not scientific and could not be proven. It still cannot be "proven," but it is no longer ignored. Researchers (e.g., Benner, 1984; Benner & Tanner, 1987) have found that experts rely on intuition a great deal at times, and frequently are right on target. Beginners also have intuition in varying degrees. Some are very tuned-in to their sixth sense; others need to nurture it for awhile. What is important for beginners is to verbalize their thoughts to someone more experienced and look for evidence to support their intuition before acting on it.

Experience

Experience is a combination of knowledge, understanding, and active participation. Even the greenest student nurse has had life experiences where he or she interacted with individuals, families, and groups. Life experience is a valuable asset in learning nursing. For each life event, coping skills are developed that may be shared with others. Experience in nursing is a key ingredient in moving from a beginner to an expert. The combination of unique life experiences and nursing experiences gives each nurse an individual style as he or she practices the art of nursing.

Self-Perception of Intelligence

In general, with the exception of close-minded egotists, the brighter a person thinks he or she is, the better that individual uses all of his or her thinking modes, and the more willing he or she is to grow in his or her thinking. It is very important for nurses to value their innate abilities, no matter how different they are from those of other nurses.

DOING IN NURSING

Doing and *thinking* are inseparable in nursing care. Knowing what one is supposed to do as a nurse will help clarify learning how to do it. Learning the *how* before developing an appreciation of the broader perspective of *what* nurses do promotes a reliance on *total recall* and *habit* modes of thinking. A learner might mimic the steps while learning nursing skills and activities, but would not appreciate how each nursing activity fits into the complex picture of great nursing.

If nurses know where they are going, they will have a better chance of engaging other thinking modes (*inquiry, new ideas and creativity, and self-awareness*) along the way. This will lead to better *doing* in the end.

Doing is the outcome of thinking in nursing. Doing is the part of nursing one can observe, the part more easily recognized; people can put labels on it. For example, nurses can be seen giving medications, making a bed, adjusting the intravenous line, teaching the patient how to change a dressing, and so forth. These doing activities are seen in real life and in the media.

Many of these tasks are often completed out of habit, but high-quality doing in nursing cannot occur without thinking. Thinking and doing are in fact so interrelated that it is difficult to separate them. It is important, however, to try to analyze each in turn so a strong base of doing knowledge can be formed to go along with the thinking knowledge.

Doing is not as simple as giving a medication or taking a blood pressure reading. Professional nursing encompasses a broad spectrum of thinking and doing activities. There are many things done that are directly related to patient care. This type of doing is called nursing interventions or nursing actions. Additionally, there are many other things that provide the background for nursing care; these are called indirect activities. Examples of these activities include patient advocacy, documenting on the patient record, and gathering data from the patient and family.

Table 6–2 and Table 6–3 provide lists of things that nurses do. Although these lists are not all inclusive, they do include most nursing care activities. The lists are divided into "direct care activities" and "indirect care activities." Distinguishing between the two categories is similar to distinguishing the categories of things nursing students do. "Direct patient care activities" are similar to going to class, studying, reading books, taking tests, and writing papers; in other words, the day-to-day student activities. Indirect student activities include registering for classes, getting bookshelves and file drawers organized, and creating a work and living situation compatible with the student role.

These lists of direct and indirect nursing activities may seem overwhelming at first glance. It takes time, practice, and a lot of thinking to master the multiple activities that nurses do.

Doing, put together with thinking, reveals how the activities fit into nursing situations. Learning skills such as how to use a sphygmomanometer to take blood pressure readings, how to prevent a patient

TABLE 6–2

A List of Direct Patient Care Activities

Caring: Conveying, through verbal and nonverbal behaviors, nurturing, supportive feelings for patients and significant others

Caretaking: Doing things for patients and their significant others that they cannot do for themselves

Counseling: Helping patients and significant others to cope more effectively with situations

Data collecting: Gathering information about the patient

Teaching: Providing information so that patients and significant others can understand to carry out activities

Implementing physician orders: Doing activities ordered by the physician as part of the medical plan of care

Monitoring: Keeping track of relevant information about the patient and the patient's situation

TABLE 6–3

A List of Indirect Patient Care Activities

Advocating: Being the patient's "agent"; looking out for his or her rights

Collaborating: Working with other health care professionals and significant others to provide care

Data collection: Gathering information about the environment around the patient and how he or she is interacting with it and significant others; sometimes this involves individual patients, at other times groups of patients

Documenting: Writing down important information about the patient

Educating self: Being a lifelong learner (even after nursing school)

Managing: Organizing and coordinating the care of several patients at once and supervising other health care workers

Referring: Connecting patients and significant others with helpful resources

Research, using, and doing: Applying new knowledge developed through systematic study and identifying areas of nursing that need further study; participating in research studies

from getting bed sores, and how to help patients cope with stress, loss, and grief, provide the content for doing. Thinking allows the nurse to know when such skills should be implemented and how those activities should be tailored to specific patient situations.

Applying Direct and Indirect Nursing Activities

To understand how direct and indirect nursing are applied to an actual patient situation, consider the following patient scenario and the accompanying discussion of how nursing care includes all of the activities listed in Tables 6–2 and 6–3.

> *Mrs. Scott cannot dress or bathe herself. She is hospitalized, status post stroke with paralysis, and confusion.*

Look at Tables 6–2 and 6–3. Think about each item on them. It is clear that caring and caretaking apply. It is likely that a nurse would be teaching Mrs. Scott adaptive ways to bathe herself. Undoubtedly, her physician would have ordered treatments and medications that the nurse would implement as well. In a hospital setting, nursing assistants often work with the nurse, so managing the part of care done by assistants also would be part of the nurse's duties.

Although there is no information on Mrs. Scott's emotional state, one could assume that she and her significant others might need some counseling to help them cope. This assumption would be based on knowledge about situational crises like strokes and how they cause stress. If the patient is to return to a healthy state, she and her significant others must cope with the stress. The nurse needs to find out how much stress this illness has precipitated. This is a good example of what was mentioned earlier; one cannot avoid thinking if one wants to do great nursing.

There are many of factors that need to be taken into account as nurses put the doing list into practice. Mrs. Scott's case illustrates the importance of considering the situation itself. A nurse needs to pay close attention to the patient in relation to where she is, how sick she is, what she wants done, when things need to be done, and many other factors. That attention means thinking.

There will be many health care providers involved in Mrs. Scott's care with whom the nurse would collaborate (other nurses; physicians; physical, occupational, and speech therapists; social workers; chaplains; dietitians and family members). Such people might automatically be part of the treatment team, or if Mrs. Scott's needs exceed the nurse's ability to intervene, the nurse might refer the patient to other health care providers, such as a home health nurse or counselor.

Often, nurses have the most consistent and frequent contact with patients and their significant others. They therefore play a key role in monitoring and noting changes in the patient's status. The nurse is frequently the advocate for the patient and significant others when their needs and the workings of the health care system are not aligned. Because nurses know the patient and the system, they use management skills to get the system to flow as smoothly as possible.

All patient situations require data collection; that is how the treatment team knows what is going on and when changes occur with the patient. Nurses need to document data, develop care plans, and monitor the results of care. Proper documentation is not only good patient care, it is required by law and institutional policies.

Every patient situation that involves a nurse is a potential research situation. Nurses need to stay abreast of the literature, reading the latest research findings and thinking about how those findings could be applied to care. Practicing nurses are also in the best position to identify gaps in the nursing knowledge base and instigate research projects.

Related to research is the need to educate oneself. Nursing and health care are changing rapidly. The primary ways to keep up on the changes are to read professional literature, go to conferences, and talk to knowledgeable people.

FACTORS INFLUENCING DOING

What nurses do is often dictated by many things other than what nursing books show as "the nursing actions" for "patient problems." Here is where thinking makes a big difference. Nurses must make decisions about how to accomplish things by evaluating all of the circumstances of a case. Each patient is an individual with a personal, subjective reality. That reality is shaped by many things, such as cultural norms, values, developmental phase of life, and many other influences.

The factors affecting how nurses do nursing are environmental, patient related, and nurse related. Obviously, it is not feasible to include all possible factors and combinations of factors in any given situation. The considerations detailed earlier are simply meant to stimulate thinking about those issues that could affect doing.

Some of these factors—specifically environmental and patient factors—are studied extensively by student nurses in courses such as psychology, sociology, and biology. The "nurse factors," however, need to be addressed because they are vital to beginning-level thinking and doing.

ASK YOURSELF

Many factors—stress, family life, lack of sleep, etc.—influence or affect how well nurses perform on any given day. What are the environmental, patient-related, and nurse-related factors that influence what you do?

Nurse Factors Influencing Doing

The first factors affecting nurses are values, beliefs, and expectations about health and health care. The best appreciation of these factors comes with self-reflection. It is possible that what people think they would feel in a given situation may not be exactly what they would feel when finally confronted with that situation. Nurses are often faced with patients who have similar or nearly identical problems, yet the surrounding circumstances make them feel differently about the situation. How do values, beliefs, and expectations influence how nurses feel or act with each patient? Are those values, beliefs, and expectations obvious to the patient because of what is said or done? Or, do values show only in subtle ways—by what is not done or said, or even by how things are said? What anyone strongly values and believes will not change overnight, but nurses should be prepared to have some of their values and beliefs challenged, and perhaps changed.

Standards, Laws, Policies, and Procedures

Standards of practice are set by state and national nursing organizations. These standards are nursing's assurance to society that a basic level of safe care will be maintained. Statements about what nurses can or cannot do are included in state nurse practice acts. Those are the laws that govern nursing practice. Each nurse should have a copy of his or her state nurse practice act for consistent and up-to-date reference. Furthermore, each institution or agency has its own set of policies and procedures that govern what nurses may do while employed at that agency. A full description of such laws, standards, policies, and procedures is beyond the scope of this chapter; however, it is essential to remember that they influence what nurses do.

Independent and Interdependent Role Functions

Nursing roles overlap with those of other health care professions, and many nursing activities are accomplished collaboratively with other health care providers. These are called interdependent nursing actions. An example of interdependent nursing actions is illustrated in the following example. After finding a patient's blood pressure to be extremely high, a nurse collaborates with the physician so that the patient's medication may be ordered or adjusted. The physician orders the medication; the nurse gives it and monitors the effects. (Except for some nurses with advanced degrees and certification, such as nurse practitioners and nurse anesthetists, nurses cannot prescribe medications.) A nurse who collaborates with the nutritionist to create an acceptable meal plan for a finicky eater on a new diabetic diet is also performing interdependent nursing actions.

Nurses exercise their independent roles when they decide what a patient needs and follow through with nursing interventions. For example, a nurse may decide independently to teach a patient how to use relaxation techniques to counteract anxiety. Or, the nurse can give a back rub to help the patient sleep better. The independent role of the nurse is based on nursing knowledge or that of another health care specialty.

Nurses use independent and interdependent actions constantly. In any given situation, a nurse may move between the two several times and do the two simultaneously. They engage their thinking skills to decide which one is appropriate at any given point. An example of the interplay between independent (I) and interdependent (ITD) nursing actions is provided in Table 6–4.

Think about how using both independent and interdependent roles helps increase the quality of care. What would be different if the nurse merely called the doctor and reported the first blood pressure reading? Would that be wrong? No, but it would be the action of a nurse with low-level thinking. The high-level thinking nurse uses both independent and interdependent actions, providing great nursing care.

Level of Expertise

Level of expertise also influences what nurses do. In some situations, nurses are very familiar with a patient's problems because they have dealt with similar situations in the past and thus have become more of an expert. In other situations it is not really apparent what should be done. Not surprisingly, beginning nursing students encounter many more of

TABLE 6–4

Example of Interaction Between Independent and Interdependent Nursing Actions

A nurse takes a patient's blood pressure and discovers that it is 160/100. This is a high reading for most people. The nurse might take any or all of the following actions:

Retake the blood pressure (I)
Observe the patient for other physical changes (I)
Ask the patient how he or she is feeling; note any changes (I)
Ask the patient what he or she was doing immediately before the blood
   pressure was taken (I)
Check the patient's record; compare previous readings to this (I)
Check the physician's order for directions related to blood pressure parameters (ITD)
Report the blood pressure reading and other findings to the physician (ITD)
Give treatment as ordered by the physician (ITD)
Monitor effects of the medication (I)
Ask the patient what he or she understands about high blood pressure and how
   it affects him or her (I)
Teach the patient relaxation techniques that might help him or her lower blood
   pressure (I)

the latter situations than the former. The scale tips in the other direction when experience is gained by nurses who keep their thinking caps on.

Much attention has been given lately to how novices and experts differ in their thinking and doing. Beginners are less likely to "know" quickly what is occurring in most patient situations. Some beginners look at experienced nurses and are amazed at how "easily" they know what to do. The stages between beginner and expert are not addressed here; one does not merely go from one to the other at some point in time. An understanding of the differences can help beginners speed up their transition to the expert level.

WAYS OF GAINING KNOWLEDGE

Beginners sometimes believe that by finding the right books to read, they will find all the answers to nursing questions and will acquire all necessary knowledge. This is not true. In the first place, there are not enough books to answer all the possible questions and provide solutions to the problems that occur in nursing situations. Secondly, the answers are always changing; what was the best answer yesterday may not be acceptable today.

Clearly, books do have useful information in them; they show what is "typical" or "standard" in many or most situations, or what a procedure ought to be like under controlled circumstances. What books cannot provide are all the possible exceptions to the "rules." That is where the thinking cap and some study skills help. By reading more than one book on the subject, one gets a new perspective. Journal articles are usually more current than books; therefore, it is a good idea to read one or two journals on a regular basis and search journals for topics of interest. Talking to experts and paying attention to one's own experience and common sense also are very helpful. Each of these strategies helps novices move beyond the beginner stage.

WAYS OF THINKING

Dualistic thinking, common for beginners, involves seeing things as only "right" or "wrong," "good" or "bad," "red" or "blue." It does not take into account the real world, where things are usually poor, good, better, or best, or shades of purple. Relativistic thinkers by contrast see the wide range of "purple" hues that make up the real world. The dualistic-thinking nurse, for example, who sees a 5-foot, 140-pound woman eating cookies might assume the patient is overweight and should not be eating cookies. The relativistic-thinking nurse by contrast might consider that the woman could be pregnant and of normal weight, could be an overweight diabetic who, incidentally, needs to eat something sweet to counteract her hypoglycemic reaction, or would at least get more information before coming to a conclusion about the merit of this person's cookie-eating behaviors (Table 6–5).

TABLE 6–5
Ways of Thinking
Dualism: Viewing knowledge as absolute and within concrete categories; information is either correct or incorrect.
Relativism: Students now begin to evaluate the different perspectives and identify possible solutions.

WAYS OF USING RULES

Context-free rules are "the steps in the book." Such steps are methods of acting or doing things without considering the unique circumstances of each patient situation. For example, when first learning how to drive a car, the beginner reads the driving manual, which says, "At a four-way stop, the person to your right gets to go through the stop first." This is a context-free rule. Although this is important to know, a driver has to consider each situation before driving through the intersection. The person to the left might be impatient and start into the intersection even though it is another driver's right to proceed first. That second driver's actions need to be adjusted to put safety first. Therefore, the rules must be interpreted in the context. The same holds true in nursing.

The following is a nursing example: Basic, context-free rules of discharge planning state: "Provide patient with written information on medications and how to take them at home." This is a good idea because written information can be used if a patient forgets what was said verbally. If that patient is illiterate or has a visual impairment, however, the written material is useless. The rule must therefore be adapted to the context of individual patient situations.

WAYS OF LOOKING AT SITUATIONS

Remember the old expression "can't see the forest for the trees"? Beginners often concentrate so hard on the pieces and details of a situation that they are unable to see that there is a larger picture. In nursing, missing the big picture is common for beginners because they have to put so much energy into keeping the details straight. For example, students giving their first injection often concentrate so hard on their technique and hitting the correct spot that they may not see other serious situations—that the patient's intravenous fluid has run out, the bed is wet, and the untouched breakfast tray is still sitting at the bedside at 3 P.M.

Does all of this mean that all beginners are doomed to think dualistically, be slaves to context-free rules or victims of narrow-mindedness? Of course not. Although these attributes are somewhat unavoidable for the new nurse, beginners will minimize their impact by engaging all thinking modes (inquiry, habits, total recall, creativity, and self-awareness) right from the start in their nursing careers. Students of nursing advance their thinking and doing as they progress through school. At the same time, it is also important to accept that no one is an expert by graduation; nurses may get there only after several years of experience. Nurses move faster along the path to expert thinking and doing when they pay attention to how they think. Thinking in all five modes helps compensate for lack of experience.

INTERTWINING DOING AND THINKING AND THE NURSING PROCESS

A goal of most nurses is to provide high-quality nursing care, or, as some would like to call it, great nursing. Achieving that goal successfully requires high-quality thinking and high-quality doing. For the beginning nurse, it is helpful to examine a simple equation that briefly illustrates *how* to achieve great nursing:

> *Patient + You + Thinking Skills + Content Knowledge*
> *+ Nursing Process = Great Nursing*

Although this greatly simplifies great nursing, it is a nice shorthand. In reality, the components are intermingled in a variety of ways.

The Patient

The **patient** may be a person, a family, a group, or a community. The usual description for nursing care with families, groups, and communities is "nursing care for aggregates." The identical nursing process is used in all cases. The big difference between using the process with individuals and using it with groups is that nurses need different content knowledge to determine what is normal and what is not normal to identify problems accurately, formulate plans, and implement and evaluate care. Table 6–6 lists a few of the different kinds of content knowledge needed to apply the nursing process.

Although interesting, a discussion of caring for aggregates is beyond the scope of this book. There is a great deal more content knowledge needed to provide effective care of families, groups, and communities. Both required and recommended books in nursing school help supply some of that information. This chapter will instead focus on the individual.

TABLE 6–6

Some Content Knowledge Needed to Apply the Nursing Process

For individuals:
- What is normal oral body temperature?
- What are typical eating patterns of 2-year-olds?
- What are the effects of chronic illness on self-esteem?

For families:
- How do members react when one person is ill?
- What happens to family roles after the first child is born?
- What are healthy family developmental stages for single-parent families?

For groups:
- What are the norms of behavior for this group?
- How cohesive is the group?
- How do the leaders of the group affect problem solving?

For communities:
- What community resources are focused on immunization clinics?
- What is the frequency of drug and alcohol use among the community's 12- to 18-year-olds?
- What health concerns are resulting from high concentrations of lead in the playground soil?

The Nurse

Every nurse is a one-of-a-kind person who hopes to be a great nurse. Each nurse's personality (feelings, values, and beliefs) as well as their thinking skills transform the basic skills acquired from textbooks into a personal art of great nursing. Using all five thinking modes helps this process.

Thinking Skills

The five thinking modes (inquiry, habits, total recall, creativity, and self-awareness) and the nurse's ability to use all of them effectively compose thinking skills. This chapter is designed to nurture and expand the reader's existing skills. Patients also have thinking skills. A major part of nursing's role is to help patients engage their thinking skills or, more generally, to help patients help themselves.

Content Knowledge

The information learned from written documents (books, journals), through interactions with others, and through nursing practice is **content knowledge**. Texts and journals contain many of the facts and concepts required during nursing school and during the remainder of one's professional career. The content knowledge from books and articles includes, for example, how illness affects coping skills; what happens to skin if a person is confined to a wheelchair and is incontinent; and all the multiple nursing needs of a teenager or elderly person with diabetes.

The other major sources of content knowledge include clinical experience and nursing research findings. It is impossible to know everything, and it is sometimes barely possible to keep current with the rapidly changing state of knowledge in health care today, but nurses must try to acquire the best content knowledge available.

The Nursing Process

Process is a way of doing something. The word "process" means moving from one point to another and changing things along the way. Many processes involve problem solving. The nursing process that includes problem solving is *how* nursing is done.

Great Nursing

This is a concept that is difficult to capture in a single definition. It is the point at which the nurse goes beyond good, safe nursing skills. Great nursing practice focuses on patients as human beings with unique strengths and unique health needs. Great nursing is creative and individualized; it is an art as well as a science.

Great nursing is not some elusive ideal that can only be aspired to and achieved in scholarly dissertations. The key to practicing great nursing is the effective use of all the components of the equation and the nurse's belief that every patient is unique.

THE NURSING PROCESS

The intertwining of thinking and doing is the nursing process. This process is the essence of professional nursing practice. The nursing process is the means by which nurses identify patients' strengths and responses to health and illness situations, design ways to assist patients in dealing with those situations, implement the needed nursing care, and determine the effectiveness of that care by looking for changes in patient behavior. Again, the nursing process is frequently a problem-solving process.

Translated into everyday language, the nursing process looks like the following: A nurse meets a patient and thinks, "What does this patient need from me, if anything?" To answer that question, the nurse considers his or her past experiences and collects some new information. The nurse thinks about what the information means, draws some conclusions about the patient's needs, and makes sure the patient agrees with those conclusions. Then the nurse thinks about and works with the patient to identify the best ways to meet the needs. The nurse performs whatever nursing care is required. After the nurse has helped the patient, the nurse and patient determine if the patient's needs have been met.

The process that the nurse goes through is similar to that used by car mechanics who must find out what is wrong with a car in order to fix it. It also is similar to the process that many others, such as hairdressers, telephone repair people, social workers, and physicians, use. Although the processes are similar for these and other groups of workers, the "focus" of each process varies. For mechanics it is car repair, for physicians it is disease curing care. For nurses it is patient care.

This process of determining what is needed and taking care of the needs may seem like common sense because it is practiced in everyday problem solving. Nursing, however, like other disciplines, has refined the basic process specifically for itself.

For many years, nurses have used specific terms to identify parts of the nursing process: *assessing, diagnosis, planning, implementing,* and *evaluating* (Figure 6–3). This chapter concentrates on thinking

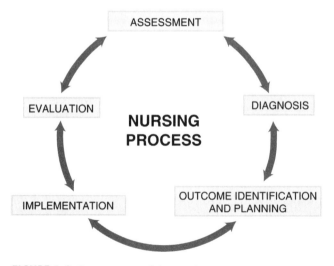

FIGURE 6–3 Components of the nursing process

and doing and on the nursing process with individuals, but, in reality, families, groups, and communities (aggregates) also are recipients of nursing care.

Definitions of the Nursing Process Components

Each of the components of the nursing process serves a special role. To understand those roles better, it is useful to examine the definitions of the components first.

Assessing

Assessment has many aspects. It is thinking about what information to collect. It is collecting information and thinking about the significance of that information. Finally, it is drawing conclusions about how the patient is responding to his or her health condition or illness. The conclusions of assessment include two basic categories: strengths and health concerns. Health concerns focus on three elements. First, issues that the nurse may deal with independently (nursing diagnosis). Next, issues that a nurse and another health care provider work on interdependently (interdisciplinary problems). Finally, issues that need to be referred to another health care provider (e.g., medical or nutrition problems).

Diagnosis

After assessing an issue, nurses break down the information and re-organize the list in terms of accepted nursing diagnoses as defined by the North American Nursing Diagnosis Association (**NANDA**). Nursing diagnoses help nurses select and plan appropriate care. Some experts, it should be noted, believe it is not necessary to include diagnosis in the nursing process because diagnosing is an integral part of assessing.

Planning

Planning is thinking about, and discussing with others, how to help with a patient's response to his or her health condition or illness. It is working with the patient in deciding which problems have priority, and in determining what the nurse and the patient need to do to meet those goals.

Implementing

Implementing is doing specific activities to help a patient meet the goals in a plan. It involves continuing to think about what is being done and how it is being done.

Evaluating

Thinking and collecting information about the patient's responses after some nursing care is provided is evaluation. It is working with the patient to determine if the patient's goals and objectives have been met and how well.

Patients and the Nursing Process

Although at times nurses do things "for" patients who cannot participate in their care, most of the time nurses work with patients collaboratively. Patients' active participation in the nursing process is a key factor of success because it indicates that patients have active roles in care. Active participation in care enhances the patient's own self-esteem and problem-solving skills. When patients are the passive recipient of care (when care is provided "for" or "to" them), they become overly dependent on the nurse and cannot achieve their optimum level of functioning.

Working "with" patients implies teamwork. The nurse asks questions, the patient responds. The patient asks questions, the nurse responds. The nurse uses thinking skills and professional judgment and comes to conclusions about the patient's strengths and health concerns. The conclusions are shared with the patient, who agrees or disagrees. If the patient agrees, the nurse and the patient plan care with specific outcomes in mind. The nurse does the nurse **doing** activities (teaching, bathing, changing dressings), and the patient does the patient activities (relaxing, exercising, washing, eating). Both evaluate the results, togetherness being the watchword.

APPLYING THE NURSING PROCESS, THINKING, AND DOING

What does the nursing process look like when applied to an individual patient? In the following case study, try to identify the components of the nursing process as well as the thinking and doing of the student nurse.

> Ms. Betty Scott, SN, is assigned to care for Mr. Mumbray, who is confined to bed with no weight-bearing on his legs. Both legs were broken when he was hit by a car one week ago. While Ms. Scott is assisting with his bed bath, she observes (assess) a pinkish-red area on his lower back. She thinks, "This is not normal. The skin over the lower back

should be the same color as the rest of the patient's skin." She next thinks, "When the skin is pink, it could mean: (1) sunburn, (2) a normal color for this patient even though it is not normal for most patients, or (3) the beginning of a pressure sore."

After asking some questions (assessing), she comes to the conclusion that this is the beginning of a pressure sore and makes the nursing diagnosis of: Impaired Skin Integrity, related to decreased circulation to the lower back secondary to immobility.

The evidence to support her nursing diagnosis (a conclusion of assessment) is:

> The skin on the patient's back is pinkish-red.
>
> This is not normal skin color for this patient's lower back.
>
> The patient has been lying on his back without turning for extended periods of time because he is confined to bed.
>
> Immobility leads to increased pressure and decreased circulation to areas of the body.
>
> Pressure and decreased circulation promote the development of pressure sores.
>
> Pressure sores are not good.

Ms. Scott develops a plan of nursing care to increase circulation and mobility, which should allow the skin to return to its usual color. She immediately implements (does) the plan, which includes explaining to the patient the importance of turning off his back at regular intervals. She writes the plan in the patient's chart so all nurses can follow it.

At the end of her shift, she checks (evaluates) to see if there is any change in the skin color on Mr. Mumbray's back and if he is turning off his back every two hours. When asked, the patient states he has been turning and there is less pinkish-red color to the skin of his lower back. Ms. Scott thinks there is good evidence to validate that she accurately identified a nursing problem and selected an appropriate intervention. She will continue to monitor Mr. Mumbray's skin for several more days.

NURSING PROCESS AND NURSING DIAGNOSES, NURSING INTERVENTIONS, AND NURSING THEORIES

Some nursing experts believe that an important addition to the original nursing process work was the development of nursing diagnosis. Until recently, there was no universal set of labels for most of the conclusions reached through assessment. Work was begun in the 1970s by a group of nurses in St. Louis, Missouri, to define more clearly the problems for which nurses provide care. The set of labels identified was called "Nursing Diagnoses." In 1976, the group expanded to an international nursing organization, the North American Nursing Diagnosis Association (NANDA). The nursing process is firmly established, the work of standardizing the terminology for nursing diagnosis is still in progress, and revisions are made every two years.

In 1992, a group of nurses in Iowa developed a set of terminology to describe what nurses do, called the "Taxonomy of Nursing Interventions." This work, like that of the NANDA group, is an attempt to define, with standard language, the realm of nursing care. The "Taxonomy of Nursing Interventions" does for implementing what the NANDA taxonomy does for assessing.

One final historical development that is important to align thinking and doing with the nursing process is the development of nursing theories. The nursing process is just what it says it is—a process; it is the *how* of nursing. But this process cannot stand alone. It needs to be combined with some framework (theory) of *what* nursing is all about. Nursing theories provide direction as to what information needs to be assessed and what to do with the information. The *how* (assessing, planning, implementing, and evaluating) is always the same, no matter what theory (framework) is used, but theories may vary in their conceptualizations of the *what* of nursing.

With all nursing theories, the nursing process remains constant, even if different terms are used to describe what nurses do. Because the nursing process can be used with just about any nursing theory, this chapter does not try to link the process specifically with one theory or another. Rather, it focuses on the process and shows how thinking and doing are inseparably intertwined throughout the process.

Brief historical highlights provide the basis for a beginning appreciation of the events and time frames of activities that have contributed to the development of the nursing process and the nursing profession. Although the formal terminology, "nursing process," is fairly recent, the problem-solving methodology used by nurses is much older. Ongoing nursing research and clinical practice continue to make giant strides in clarifying and refining the use of the nursing process in the continuous improvement of nursing.

Part of the ongoing task of a socially responsible profession is to continue to define and describe clearly what it does for the protection and safety of the public. The continuous process of refining, clarifying, labeling, and developing standards of care, although necessary, is a double-edged sword. Definitions, descriptions, and standards are professional mandates, they also carry with them the danger of making nursing appear to have cookbook-type recipes for care.

Some nurses strongly criticize the use of any labels or standardized approaches. The major criticisms are based on two beliefs. First, attempts to label and standardize care are too simplistic for the uniqueness of individuals and their needs. Second, the dynamic nature of people, their environment, and nursing care are too complex to infer any direct cause-and-effect relationship between nursing care and the results of care.

In most cases, however, it is not standardized approaches that are at fault, but rather what is done with those approaches when they are used as cookbook recipes, devoid of much thought. Unfortunately, the thinking and the necessity for focusing attention on the individual can be lost along the road to defining and standardizing terminology and approaches.

A standardized approach, like the nursing process, is similar to a cake recipe. The recipe works fine if the cook has all the correct ingredients in all the correct amounts, the correct size pan, and the correct oven temperature. But what happens if one ingredient is missing? Can some other ingredient be substituted? What happens if the oven doesn't get as hot as the recipe calls for? Can a lower temperature be used, or is it better simply to bake the cake longer? Without the ability to think and make adjustments in the recipe, the result will be something much different than the desired cake. The thinking cook, however, can modify the recipe and still end up with a great cake.

The same principle applies in nursing. Standards and labels are only guides; the nurse must think and adjust standards and labels to fit each patient's unique needs. Thinking provides the nurse and the patient with multiple avenues to achieve the same goal. It is continually necessary for both beginning nurses and experienced nurses to keep those thinking caps on and avoid the rut of cookbook nursing.

The skills the nurse must have in order to use the nursing process are intellectual, interpersonal, and technical. Intellectual skills entail problem solving, critical thinking, and making nursing judgments. Nursing is in continuous transition, and there is still much to do. Part of what is exciting is that the nursing leaders, who will guide thinking and doing and the nursing process into the twenty-first century, are the beginning nurses of today.

SEQUENCING THE NURSING PROCESS COMPONENTS

With the recognition that the nursing process and thinking and doing are the foundation of successful practice comes the question, "Where does the process start?" Consider the following clinical situation:

> A student nurse is assigned to care for a female patient for the morning. The patient is 85, very independent, and does not like to bother people. Today she is confined to bed after her hip surgery yesterday. The student nurse walks into her room and finds her struggling to complete her bed bath even though she can't reach the lower part of her legs. What is the first thing to consider?

If the nurse states, "I need to help the patient finish her bath," he or she is thinking about implementing first. If the nurse says, "I need to get some information about the patient first," then he or she is thinking about assessing. Others might say, "I need to sit down and decide what is the best way to help this patient. Should I do it myself, or find another way to help her finish the task so she doesn't have to give up her independence?" The nurse is approaching this from the point of planning (Table 6–7).

As with most of nursing, there is no absolute right or wrong place to start. Although thinking may focus on any component of the nursing process first, the most logical doing starts with assessment. Logically, if the nurse has never seen the patient before, some information (assessment) is needed before doing anything if safe nursing care is to be achieved. All encounters begin with some degree of assessment. How much information is needed depends on other circumstances, such as how immediate the patient's need is (severe bleeding, not breathing), how much experience the nurse has (beginner or expert), and how

TABLE 6–7

Thinking Questions: Assessment Through Planning

Assessment
- What does the information mean?
- What information is available? Is there a nursing problem?
- Does the information support the problem?
- Are there any other influencing factors?
- What is the conclusion?
- Does the conclusion make sense to the patient?

Planning
- How does the problem's priority compare to other health concerns?
- What is the goal for this problem?
- Does the goal make sense?
- What are the expected outcomes?

More Inquiry Thinking
- Should the problem be ignored or referred?
- Is the problem really a nursing problem?
- Is a collaborative effort needed?
- What are the available resources?

much time is available to spend with the patient (ten minutes during an office visit or many months in a nursing home).

Similar circumstances will influence how much time and energy nurses put into planning care. Sometimes planning is instantaneous, on the spot. Other times the nurse can sit for an hour or two and write a lengthy, long-term plan of care. Likewise, implementation may vary depending on the situation. Evaluation always occurs after something is done. It does not make much sense to try to evaluate changes in patient behaviors before any care is provided.

In any given patient encounter, nurses may assess, plan, implement, and evaluate several times as well as use all the components at the same time. The nurse may also spend varying amounts of time and energy on each component of the process. Consider these examples: (1) the nurse may assess for a new problem (e.g., diaper rash) while evaluating care outcomes for an old problem (e.g., how well Mom learned to diaper the baby); (2) likewise, as the nurse implements care for a patient's problem (e.g., turning a patient on his side to relieve pain), the nurse may assess for other concerns (e.g., skin conditions, mobility) and even evaluate the results of care for another problem (e.g., how well the patient has learned to use the trapeze to help with moving in bed) while planning care for yet another problem (e.g., the best toileting schedule). And, believe it or not, this may be accomplished in several seconds by more experienced nurses. Although it may take a little longer for beginning nurses, the same events in thinking and doing will occur if the nursing process is used effectively.

The "bottom line" is that there are four key components to the nursing process. All four are critical to high-quality nursing care, and all four are used repeatedly for each nursing concern. Where to start and how much emphasis to place on each component at a certain point in care depend on many factors, including the patient situation, the nurse's expertise, and the amount of time available. Some degree of assessment, even if it only takes microseconds, is usually the starting point.

THINKING INTO THE FUTURE

Knowing the five modes of thinking (inquiry, habits, total recall, creativity, and self-awareness) is the foundation for critical thinking and sound clinical judgment. Clearly understanding the multiple roles of direct and indirect care activities helps define the domain of what nurses do, and appreciating the intertwining of thinking and doing with the multiple processes within the nursing process is necessary to move beyond the role of beginner.

It is the growing level of comfort and ease in using all five modes of thinking skills that is of particular importance. To broaden one's perspective on thinking, it is wise to consider these thinking skills as more than separate entities. The five modes work in harmony with each other all at the same time. Compare the modes of thinking to the strings on a guitar: Each mode, like each string has its own special purpose, but when all the strings are used together to play a piece of music, the result is much nicer than if just one or two strings were played alone. The same idea applies to the use of the thinking modes. The more they are used in harmony with each other, the better the result.

The five modes of thinking are integral parts of the patient as well as the nurse. Thinking skills are developed over time and can be enhanced for both nurse and patient.

Self-awareness is the key mode for nurturing the growth of all thinking modes for both the nurse and the patient. Some refer to this mode as "reflective thinking." Reflective thinking has been studied for over a decade. Critical thinking competencies include:

- Interpretation: Categorizing, decoding, and clarifying meaning
- Analysis: Examining ideas, identifying arguments, analyzing arguments, and identifying implications, possible complications, and possible relationships
- Evaluation: Assessing information and responses
- Inference: Questioning evidence; drawing conclusions based on evidence
- Explanation: Stating results; justifying procedures
- Self-regulation: Continuously monitoring, reflecting on, and questioning one's own thinking

There is never an end to the learning of content knowledge. What is learned today may be different tomorrow, or maybe even in a few minutes. Great nursing is impossible if nurses stop learning content knowledge.

Nurses must also know about the activities of other health professionals to effectively identify, collaborate on, and refer health concerns. The major content knowledge required of nurses, besides nursing knowledge, is in the biomedical field. Although many expert nurses are sophisticated enough in their content knowledge to determine medical diagnoses, it is not within the legal realm of nursing practice to make medical diagnoses.

The purpose of having strong content knowledge in the biomedical field is not to make medical diagnoses but to supplement nursing practice. For example, a patient with all the signs and symptoms of diabetes can be identified by the nurse and referred to the physician for the official diagnosis. The nurse then diagnoses the many possible and probable nursing needs of the patient, who must manage the activities of daily living affected by the disease. The nurse determines how the diabetes is affecting sleep patterns, activity patterns, eating patterns, skin care, and so forth. All of those effects of the disease become the human responses for which nurses are responsible as they diagnose and design care.

The sources of content knowledge are expanding. Lectures, workshops, books, journals, computer searches, other health professionals, patients, significant others, and experience are only some of the many sources of information.

The strong connections between content knowledge and thinking become obvious as the nurse looks for the many possible and probable relationships among the multiple content areas: the patient's individual responses to the situation at hand; the patient's strengths and resources; what the nurse knows or needs to look up about health and illness; the domain of nursing; and the domain of other health care professionals.

Great nursing continues to be a concept that is not easy to describe precisely and clearly. Great nursing is usually easy to recognize in action, but it is elusive to pin down with words. Consider the following comparison of adequate nursing to great nursing to help make the distinction clearer:

> *Adequate nursing care:* Safe care because all parts of the nursing process are used. (Unsafe, poor nursing care is the result of skipping one or more of the parts.) The nurse who provides adequate care mechanically plods through all the components of the nursing process in a series of separate steps that simply follow each other in a linear fashion. The primary thinking modes used are *total recall* and *habits.*

> *Great nursing care:* Safe, efficient, and effective care that results from using the nursing process as the dynamic tool it was designed to be. Assessing, planning, implementing, and evaluating are done by nurses using all modes of thinking. The nursing process becomes embedded into the nurse's thinking process. The nursing process is no longer a separate entity that requires retrieval from a textbook or even from conscious memory during each patient encounter. Care is focused on the patient as a unique individual. When nursing is great, it is a caring art as well as a sophisticated science (Figure 6–4).

The future holds many challenges for nursing and nurses. For example, technology threatens to depersonalize both the patient and the nurse while it leads nursing into the new age. Cost-containment measures are eliminating nursing positions, while, at the same time, they force the use of *new ideas* and *creativity* to find better ways to deliver great care. Proposals for new national health care policies are seen as threats by some and blessings by others. One predicted conse-

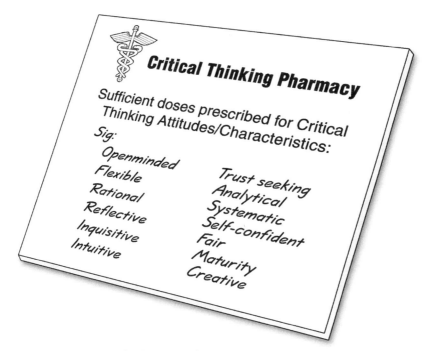

Critical Thinking Pharmacy

Sufficient doses prescribed for Critical
Thinking Attitudes/Characteristics:

Sig:

Openminded
Flexible
Rational
Reflective
Inquisitive
Intuitive

Trust seeking
Analytical
Systematic
Self-confident
Fair
Maturity
Creative

FIGURE 6–4 Critical thinking attitudes

quence of national policy change is a significant increase in the need for nurses to be primary providers of service to many populations.

Change is guaranteed and the best any nurse can do is to be prepared. Great nursing is not an elusive ideal that may only be written about by nursing scholars. Great nursing is practiced hourly by nurses in all health care settings, including homes, long-term care facilities, schools, clinics, intensive care units, urgent care clinics, and hospitals, to name only a few. Great nursing is even practiced by student nurses as they incorporate the components of the equation into their practice.

The Ideal Critical Thinker

The ideal critical thinker is habitually inquisitive, well-informed, trust-ful of reason, open-minded, flexible, fair-minded in evaluation, honest in facing personal biases, prudent in making judgments, willing to reconsider, clear about issues, orderly in complex matters, diligent in seeking relevant information, reasonable in the selection of criteria, focused in inquiry, and persistent in seeking results that are as precise as the subject and the circumstances of inquiry permit.

KEY POINTS

- Patient care includes direct patient care activities and indirect patient care activities.
- The nurse factors affecting doing include values, beliefs, and expectations; standards, laws, policies, and procedures; role functions; and the level of expertise.
- The five modes of thinking are total recall, habits, inquiry, new ideas and creativity, and knowing how you think.
- Great nursing results from using the nursing process as the dynamic tool it was designed to be.

 CASE STUDY

Jerry, A student nurse, is completing a day on a busy surgical unit. At 10 A.M., he had just completed a bed bath for one of his patients. He then went to the medication room to prepare the medications for his three patients. Just before he finished this, the charge nurse told him that the patient in Room 8, Mr. Norris, was requesting a pain medication. Jerry saved some time and prepared the 10 mg of morphine ordered for the patient. He gathered the medications he had prepared, and went to Room 8 first, giving Mr. Jones his ordered medications and then giving Mr. Norris the requested injection of morphine. After administering all the medications, Jerry looked at Mr. Norris' chart and discovered that he had received morphine only two hours before. The medication is to be given no more often than every four hours. Within 15 minutes of receiving the morphine, Mr. Norris' vital signs were stable. As a follow-up, Jerry completed an incident report describing the medication error.

Evaluate this experience while considering the errors that were made and describe what Jerry might learn from the experience.

CRITICAL THINKING ACTIVITIES

Select a recently assigned patient. Reflecting on your actions during that experience, prepare an outline that describes your plan of care for future patients with similar health care needs. As you complete the plan, consider these questions: What might you do differently? What might you do in the same way? How might you improve the patient's participation in your plan?

BIBLIOGRAPHY

Barnum, B. S. (1994). Realities in nursing practice: A strategic view. *Nursing and Healthcare, 15*(8), 400–405.

Boston, C., & Vestal, K. W. (1994). Work transformation. *Hospitals and Health Networks, 68*(7), 50–54.

Catalano, J. C. (1994). A survey of educators' activities to empower nurses for practice. *Nursing Outlook, 42*(4), 182–187.

Costelle-Nickitas, D. M. (1997). Get ready to take charge. *American Journal of Nursing, 97*(5), 16B–16J.

Rocchiccioli, J., & Tilbury, M. (1998). *Clinical leadership in nursing.* Philadelphia: W. B. Saunders.

Sullivan, E., & Decker, P. (1997). *Effective leadership and management in nursing* (4th ed.). Menlo Park, CA: Addison-Wesley.

INTERNET RESOURCES

Citizen's Council on Health Care
http://www.cchc-mn.org
Health hotlines
http://www.cdcnac.org/sis
Health on the Net
http://www.hon.ch
Hospital Web
http://neuro-www.mgh.harvard.edu/hospitalweb.shtml
Support Resources
http://www.cmhc.com/sxlist.htm

CHAPTER **7**

Leadership and Management in Nursing

OVERVIEW

Today many events are changing the role of the nurse manager. Never before has there been such a need for nurses to work competently and collaboratively with other health care professionals to secure cost-effective quality health care for all. Nurses must be skilled leaders and competent managers in the new health care environment. This chapter explores how nurses as leaders and managers enhance the delivery of quality health care. Ideally, leaders and managers possess a vision that energizes the group and calls forth the best efforts of members. As critical thinkers and responsible decision makers, they commit high energy to goal achievement and are skilled in enlisting support and cooperation.

OBJECTIVES

Upon completion of this chapter, the reader should be able to:

- Define the differences between leadership and management.
- Describe the four components of the management process.
- Identify three skills required for effective management.
- Characterize leadership and management functions of common nursing roles.
- Identify and describe three models of nursing care delivery.
- Describe four types of power and describe the role of power in leadership and management.

⇒ KEY TERMS

Controlling	Management
Directing	Organizing
Leadership	Planning

INTRODUCTION

Leaders value learning and must be knowledgeable. They understand that it is impossible to be an expert about all aspects of the profession. Therefore, they develop and use resources. A good manager fosters an environment that empowers employees to make decisions independently. This leaves the nurse manager free to act as a link between nurses and upper management.

LEADERSHIP VS. MANAGEMENT

What is the difference between leadership and management? Many people do not feel there is a significant distinction. Leadership and management often blend together without a clear concept of their unique and powerful differences; however, it is important to understand these distinct concepts.

Broadly defined, **leadership** is the ability to influence others, often toward a particular goal or vision. Leadership is often characterized as charisma, but this is not quite correct. It is also a skill set that may be learned. **Management**, by contrast, is a systematic process similar in some respects to the nursing processes. It emphasizes problem solving and implementing solutions. A few management traits are planning, organizing, and prioritizing.

At the institutional level, leadership abilities and management skills are required to provide the circumstances in which nurses can practice. At the individual nurse-patient level, leadership and good management skills are required to determine the plan of nursing care, integrate that plan of care effectively with other health care professionals, and coordinate the interdisciplinary treatment plan for the client.

Although most nurses are clinicians, education and management roles exist in most organizations where nurses practice to provide the education, management, communication, and representation required for nurses to practice nursing.

These definitions should begin to clarify the differences between leadership and management. It is important to recognize, however, that this is a gross simplification. There is no one best way (or one best set of behaviors) for effective leadership or management. Research indicates that different leaders and managers have different inherent traits and abilities. A leader's effectiveness depends not only on his or her traits, skills, and behaviors, but also on characteristics of the followers and factors in the situation, such as their shared purpose and desire for change.

LEADERSHIP

Effective leadership occurs when a person with the right combination of personality traits and abilities applies those skills to the appropriate circumstances. A leader who is successful in one situation may not be as successful in another.

Leadership Skills

There are four basic skill sets that all nursing leaders possess to varying degrees. These skills help leaders achieve the goals and objectives that an organization may have.

Communication

Leaders—especially nurses—need to possess the ability to build trusting interpersonal relationships. This is as important for peers, staff, and superiors as it is for patients. Open and honest communication helps organizations maximize goals and enhance the personal growth of all participants.

Problem Solving

Nurses are natural problem solvers. This is fortunate because leaders spend much of their time searching for solutions. They need to be able to analyze all sides of a problem, to explore multiple options, and to work to a creative solution. The ability to plan, implement, and stabilize change are a key to problem solving.

Delegation

Good leaders do not do everything themselves. The ability to direct others toward organizational goals is essential. It involves recognizing and fostering the unique talents and skills of others and the ability to match these skills with necessary tasks. Delegators need organizational and financial skills as well as the ability to manage resources.

Self-Evaluation

Leaders should be able to honestly assess their effectiveness. This includes taking blame as well as praise. Acknowledging faults allows for future improvements.

Leadership Styles

In addition to the established leadership skills, there are several identified leadership styles. It is important to know and understand them. Both employees and managers need to recognize their own particular leadership style. Each nurse should understand his or her own predominant style and reinforce or alter it depending on its effectiveness. This allows employees and managers to work well with different managers.

Research has identified four styles of leadership in managers from various fields, not just nursing. These styles range from directive to participative, depending on the amount of staff participation in decision making. They are autocratic, democratic, laissez-faire, and participative.

Autocratic

An autocratic leader is typically task oriented. He or she tends to make decisions independently. Little or no input is sought from the larger group. This leader feels he or she is in complete control. Although this may sound terrible, there are advantages in having an autocratic leader. The classic example is in an emergency, when there is no time to delay (Table 7–1).

TABLE 7–1

Working with Autocratic Leaders

- Autocratic leaders are free with both praise and criticism.
- The instructions provided are not hidden or subtle.
- These leaders usually respond well in an emergency.
- The group does not participate in group decision making.

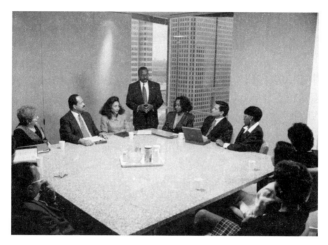

FIGURE 7–1 A democratic leader asks for input from the team during a brainstorming session. *(Courtesy of Photodisc)*

Democratic

A democratic leader is focused on the individual characteristics and abilities of each staff member. He or she strives to secure consensus and commitment to their decisions. This leader tries to empower employees, encouraging them to establish their own goals. These traits are often appealing to most staff because the individual is well represented in all activities of the organization (Figure 7–1).

Most people are initially drawn to the democratic leader. They like the individual attention this type of leader provides and enjoy being part of a team; however, sometimes members of a group leave this type of leader because of the time-consuming process of making decisions.

Democratic leaders need to know when to lead. Not all decisions require or should involve employees (Table 7–2).

TABLE 7–2
Working with Democratic Leaders

- There is a time commitment in working with the group process.
- There are few secrets kept from the group.
- Emergencies within this leadership environment are stressful, especially if a decision needs to be made quickly.

ASK YOURSELF

Leadership and You

If you were to categorize the type of leadership that allows you to do your best work, what would it be? Do you seek the honesty and directness of the autocratic leader, thrive on the group discussions of the democratic leader, need the autonomy of the laissez-faire leader, or gain confidence and professional strength working with a participative leader? Each leadership style has its advantages and inherent disadvantages and you need to identify the ones that support you in your professional growth and endeavors.

Laissez-faire

The laissez-faire leader is often referred to as the "let alone" leader. This person overemphasizes delegation to the point of neglecting their leadership responsibilities. This leaves employees without direction, supervision, or coordination in their projects. Because there is no strong leader to organize and manage group work, the staff often decides on its priorities.

Many people avoid working with a laissez-faire leader because of the lack of guidance, caring, and instructions. Those who do work in a laissez-faire environment are often out of touch with the rest of the organization, because the manager does not pass information efficiently (Table 7–3).

Participative

The multicratic or participative leader is a compromise between the autocratic and democratic leadership styles. This leader analyzes problems and develops solutions and then presents them to the larger

TABLE 7–3

Working with Laissez-faire Leaders

- This person provides minimum guidance, information.
- This work environment provides a great deal of autonomy.
- There is a danger of chaos owing to the lack of information.
- The staff may be out of synchrony with the rest of the organization.

TABLE 7–4

Working with Participative Leaders

- The group generally has an active role in decision making.
- Relatively little information is kept from members of the group.
- There is a free exchange of ideas.

group. He or she then invites criticism and comments. This leader listens to employee feedback but makes all final decisions independently. This person works well both within the group and in an emergency when matters must be handled immediately.

This type of leader provides many advantages for workers in this situation. Confidence emanates from him or her to both management and staff. It allows the staff to share their ideas freely with the leader and contribute to the goal-setting process in a significant manner. A final point is that control and power are widely spread throughout the group because of this style of leadership (Table 7–4).

Licensed Practical/Vocational Nursing Leadership

Many people in the health care environment argue that leadership and management roles are not appropriate for the Licensed Practical/Vocational Nurse (LPN/LVN). Those people should walk down the hallway of any nursing home or hospital in this country. A tour of these facilities is powerful evidence that LPN/LVNs not only need to take a leadership role, but that it already has been taken by LPN/LVNs.

LPN/LVNs exhibit leadership in many ways. They are managers of care for patients. They are advocates for patients and resources within the health care system. It is important to note, however, that an LPN/LVN is required to practice under both the state's nurse practice act and the supervision of a registered nurse (RN). Nevertheless, LPN/LVNs are assuming many leadership roles with the encouragement of the health care system.

One of the many reasons for this change was the work redesign of many health care organizations. Under the constant pressure to reduce costs and provide affordable health care, many administrators began exploring all avenues for saving. One of the most significant changes was the hiring of LPN/LVNs to replace RNs, depending on the patient care delivery system employed by individual health care facilities. This was a dramatic change.

LPN/LVNs are now often required to assume management responsibilities in with other LPN/LVNs and multiskilled paraprofessional
workers such as nurse assistants. Some LPN/LVNs are employed as
directors of nursing, a definite leadership role. This is in addition to
their historic role as both managers and leaders in long-term care facilities where, with an administrator's license, they may be employed as
administrators. There are now many opportunities for LPN/LVNs to
assume the role of leader and manager. These roles will only increase.

ROLE TRANSITION

Too often, professional nurses in any health care setting receive little
formal management training before being promoted to the management team. It is the nurse's education that ultimately facilitates the role
transition to manager. Once a nurse is promoted, it is thought that
some skills may have to be changed or even unlearned. The challenge
is to provide new managers with the information and skills needed to
develop fundamental and successful behaviors and thought processes
that effectively contribute to work accomplishment.

Luckily, most new nurse managers bridge parts of this gap using the
clinical and educational experiences they bring to the new position.
These skills are what nurses do well every day and include communicating, planning, organizing, prioritizing, and documenting. All are
talents that lend themselves well to the new role of nurse manager.
Further expansion into the nurse manager role is based on learned
management behaviors including planning, organizing, directing,
controlling, and evaluating.

The nurse manager's orientation should follow a formal plan. It is
important to note that no program, however well thought out, can
address all the issues that will confront the new nurse manager in any
setting. Some skills develop fully only after a period of time with the
integration of knowledge and practice. These good habits become
"automatic" only with use.

Formal and Informal Leaders

There is a great deal of material written about the concept of leadership. Everyone acknowledges that it is desirable to have a strong leader
in an organization. In every hospital, department, and organization,

there is an office, a nameplate, and often a secretary, which indicate a formal environment. In health care this person may have the title of administrator or president. Yet there are many more opportunities for leadership, and focusing on a formal position hides many excellent ways for LP/VNs to apply and grow their leadership skills.

The Formal Leader

The formal leader is easily recognizable as such. He or she often does not interact with patients or give them care. Sometimes they do not even interact frequently with the caregivers. The responsibility of the assigned leader is to anticipate the changes in health care systems and to lead the organization to a comfortable or successful place in that future awareness or vision. This is the person who should know when to expand an organization and when to cut the caseload.

Most organizations have leaders on another level. This could be a nurse manager in a hospital or long-term care facility, or a case manager in a home health agency. These leaders are accountable to the higher level administrator or president, but have their domain to lead. This again is a formal leader; someone who has a title, a name tag, and generally an office. This formal leader may or may not provide patient care, but definitely does frequently interact with the caregivers.

The Informal Leader

The other type of leader is the informal leader. This is a role that even the recent graduate can fill. There is no official title or office. Instead, it is a person on the care team who is respected because of his or her insight, drive, or passion.

The informal leader does not prepare the schedule or determine the raises but instead works within the assigned workload. He or she is easily identified within the group. It is the individual everyone looks to when a decision has to be made or when a controversial topic is discussed. This person leads by example, building morale and energizing coworkers.

An effective formal leader looks for, identifies, and respects informal leaders. Informal leaders have power with the group, expertise in patient care, and the ability to lead the group in the direction of the formal leader's choice. A wise formal leader quickly develops a positive working relationship with the informal leaders in the organization.

TABLE 7–5

Economic and Professional Issues That Affect the Work Environment

Economic Issues
- Increases in number of patients without health insurance
- More acutely ill patients seeking care
- Third-party payer restrictions on covered care
- Spiraling costs of health care

Professional Issues
- Ethical dilemmas
- Redesign of organizations and change in patient care delivery model
- Values clarification
- Rotation and weekend work, on call, other staffing needs
- "Quicker and sicker" syndrome causing staff to respond by "doing the best they can"
- Managed care
- Customer service focus
- Outcomes management
- The need for more collaborative and interdisciplinary relationships
- Professional development/continuing education
- Staff, patient, and provider diversity issues

THE MANAGEMENT ENVIRONMENT

All nurse managers face economic and professional influences that affect their work environment. These may be internal in the organization or external in the larger health care environments. Some of the most important contemporary influences are listed in Table 7–5.

MANAGEMENT

Management is getting a job done or accomplishing a goal by planning, organizing, directing, and controlling. In any setting, these four management functions provide a way to organize people, things, and activities, and to direct them toward overall objectives. These management functions provide the glue that holds the organization together. In health care organizations, managers must organize the health care professionals and support staff; the building space, supplies, and equipment; and the client care and support activities. The four management functions help accomplish the overall objective of providing quality client care.

Management is all about organization. It is the ability to organize details so organizational goals may be successfully achieved. The manager is often seen as the person who is responsible for getting work done through others. This requires excellent interpersonal relationship skills; broad understanding of the organization and how it works; and the ability to perceive the organization as patient focused, to establish goals and objectives, to utilize manpower and physical plant resources, and to act as an agent of change.

Functions of Managers

All nurses are leaders. Some nurses, because of their positions in the health care system, are also managers. The role of the nurse manager is to plan, organize, direct, and control available resources to deliver quality care to patients and families. These management functions— planning, organizing, directing, and controlling—help accomplish the overall objective of providing quality client care and each will be discussed separately.

Planning

Planning is deciding what to do, when, where, how, by whom, and with what resources. It is an ongoing process that involves assessing, setting goals, establishing priorities, developing action plans, and evaluating whether the actions are meeting the objectives. Planning provides direction for the people involved, meaning for the work activities, and a scheme for efficient use of the people, space, and equipment.

In a nursing department, the top-level manager, the nurse executive, devotes a great deal of time to planning. He or she outlines the department's goals and determines the numbers and types of nurses and other personnel required to provide those services. In contrast, the department's lowest-level manager, the staff nurse, devotes less time to planning. This nurse assesses each patient and determines needs, sets priorities, and develops a plan for nursing care. The plan of care answers the questions of what we do, when, where, and how.

Organizing

The challenge of **organizing** is breaking down work into small units so it may be readily accomplished. It also involves setting expectations, determining responsibilities, and establishing lines of communication and reporting relationships. The nurse executive ensures that the department has objectives that match priorities. He or she also details job descriptions that assign responsibilities and reporting relationships. The nurse executive often delegates to others the responsibility and accountability for much of the work. For example, the responsibility for direct nursing care is delegated to staff nurses.

The staff nurse organizes patient care by establishing the goals, interventions (things to be done), and expected outcomes of the care. The plan of care, nursing documentation, and nursing shift report communicate priorities to other nurses who are delegated responsibility for delivering some of the nursing care.

Directing

Directing involves supervision and ongoing decision making. Work tasks are assigned, instructions provided, expectations are communicated, and guidance is provided. The nurse executive directs much of the change for the department by supervising the next level managers; he or she devotes much less time to directing than to planning and controlling.

The charge nurse directs the work of the shift by assigning patients, scheduling meal breaks and times, and determining who will admit and care for patients admitted during the shift. The staff nurse directs the care for patients by ordering nursing care, communicating the care on the written plan of care and in shift reports, and supervising the care delivered by others.

Controlling

Controlling is verifying that plans are in fact carried out as planned. It also includes evaluating staff. Some steps in the control process are measuring results against preestablished standards or expectations and taking action to reinforce effective actions and to change ineffective ones.

The nurse executive monitors the results of recruitment, staff turnover, and budget performance against expectations. He or she uses the performance appraisal process to acknowledge positive performance and to promote further growth in staff. The staff nurse reassesses the patient to determine whether the prescribed nursing interventions and interdisciplinary treatments are resulting in patient improvement, whether interventions need to be changed, and whether other interventions should be added.

Management Skills

Managers bring a host of innate skills and abilities to their role. These, to varying degrees, help managers attain organizational objectives. Because managers deal with people, ideas, and things, the effective manager must be skilled in problem solving, communicating, and managing change.

Problem Solving

Problem solving is a systematic process that involves several steps. First, the problem must be identified and analyzed. Next, possible solutions need to be proposed. The consequences of each possible outcome must be considered and a solution selected. Finally, the solution may be implemented. Ultimately, the results will also need to be evaluated. Throughout the process, all departments involved in the issues must be continuously identified and included. This allows for appropriate input from all areas in the organization that may be affected by the issue and the possible outcomes.

Communication

Communication is a prerequisite to problem solving and one of the fundamental skills of management. Research shows that managers spend 75 to 90 percent of their time communicating in one form or another with others. Staff nurses also spend a large amount of their time communicating with patients, families, other nurses, physicians, and other health care professionals and support staff.

Managers must have effective writing, speaking, and listening skills. The sender must be able to translate desires into a form that the receiver can understand. The interpretation of the message may be influenced by several factors such as differences in the sender's and receiver's skills, background experiences, education, trust, values, semantics, and emotional states. The status differences between the manager and staff also may affect communication effectiveness.

The nonverbal cues accompanying the message are essential aspects of verbal communication. If the sender's tone, speed, inflection of voice, facial expression, or other nonverbal behaviors are consistent with the verbal message, communication will be enhanced; however, if any of these are inconsistent with the verbal message, the receiver will believe the nonverbal message instead of the verbal one.

Listening is an important part of effective verbal communication. It may be hampered by the listener's lack of interest in the topic, premature interpretation of the message, or preoccupation with preparing a response. Good listening is a choice of actions that can be improved with practice. To be more effective the listener should (1) give full attention to what the speaker is saying; (2) listen to the facts and feelings; (3) avoid formulating a response or judging the meaning until the speaker has finished; (4) use questions to clarify meanings.

Communication skills are necessary for successful implementation of the management process. Managers depend on communication to stay informed, to assist with planning and decision making, and to convey decisions to others. Effective leaders inspire staff by successfully communicating a shared meaning of goals, direction, and vision. Staff nurses rely on communication to care for patients and families, to relate to coworkers, and to function as effective interdisciplinary team members.

Legal Aspects of Management

One of the most essential aspects of management is an understanding of the law. Nurses are generally responsible for the acts and omissions of all of the practitioners they supervise. Their liability is based on legal theory called *respondeat superior*, which literally means "let the master say." The theory is that because supervisors control what practitioners do, they are therefore legally responsible for their errors.

The only exception to this rule occurs when, despite appropriate supervision, practitioners take it upon themselves to do something that is entirely outside the scope of their job functions. A classic example of this conduct involves nurses who voluntarily provide care to patients in their homes after they have been discharged from the hospital, facility, or home health agency. As long as management is able to demonstrate that a policy was established that prohibited this conduct, liability for injuries to patients during such "detours" may rest solely with the practitioners.

Questions of appropriate delegation to certain types of practitioners are controlled almost exclusively by state laws. That is, state licensure statutes govern which functions related to patient care may be delegated to certain types of practitioners. Nurse managers must thoroughly understand these statutes in the states in which their organization provides services in order to ensure that functions are properly delegated. Any questions or areas of uncertainty should be referred to the appropriate state licensure boards for written clarification.

Many nurse managers are understandably concerned about the scope of their responsibilities for everyone who falls within their chain of command. They certainly cannot provide direct supervision to each practitioner they supervise on a daily basis. This valid concern serves to reinforce the importance of hiring and retaining practitioners who provide care to patients in an appropriate manner. It also underscores the need to take prompt disciplinary action with regard to practitioners who do not meet established standards.

Even though every practitioner's actions cannot be supervised directly, significant legal issues exist that always merit the attention of competent nurse managers. New managers should immediately focus their attention on these issues and continuously monitor developments in the areas of negligence, employment, and consent to treatment.

Importance of Policies

Policies and procedures constitute perhaps the most important source for standards of care. Developing appropriate standards of care through policies and procedures is certainly a double-edged sword for nurse managers. Although it provides an opportunity to establish standards that are appropriate for institutions and staff members, the law requires strict adherence to these standards once they have been developed.

In addition, developing policies and procedures is an exceptionally tedious task for several reasons. First, some nurses believe that policies and procedures should cover every possible contingency associated with the policy subject. Nurses who share this belief want such policies so that they feel they have clear guidance. Other nurses, however, believe that policies and procedures should provide only broad guidance, within which nurses should exercise appropriate professional judgment. Obviously, finding a balance between these two competing goals is necessary. Policies that are too detailed often prove useless because staff members do not have the time or inclination to read through volumes to understand procedures. Conversely, promoting clarity or expectations of staff members is one of the basic tenets of effective nursing management.

Developing standards of care is further complicated by the sheer number of individuals and committees that review new or revised policy or procedure. Often, what goes into the process bears little resemblance to the final result. Despite these obstacles, nurse managers must persist in developing and maintaining appropriate policies and procedures. A key to success is to avoid thinking that this process is ever complete. Nursing policies and procedures should be under almost constant review and scrutiny; they are not static. Rather, they

TABLE 7–6
Reducing Risk Through Policies and Procedures

- Review policies and procedures at least annually.
- Involve different staff members in reviews so various points of view are obtained.
- Make needed changes promptly.
- Ensure that all staff members are informed of changes in policies and procedures.
- Ensure that all new staff members read and understand the policies and procedures.

change often because of experience, judgment, and new clinical developments (Table 7–6).

Delegation

Delegation is a very critical issue. As hospitals instituted nursing care models that included unlicensed assistive personnel, the need for delegation grew. It emerged as a means to meet the demands of the nursing shortage and a method to control or cut the cost of providing primary care when nursing salaries rose and reimbursement dropped.

The new nurse manager must realize that there are different health care providers who can safely and effectively provide care to patients if they function within the constraints of their state or natural scope of practice and protocols of care. Using unlicensed personnel to assist with those elements of patient care (e.g., bed baths, feeding, venipuncture) frees trained nursing staff for patient care. The important elements for both nursing staff and management are the training and credentialing of the unlicensed staff member. These staff members, similar to the home health aide in home care, are integral and useful and can bring new perspectives to the care planning process; however, their practice needs to be structured, supervised, and delegated appropriately (Figure 7–2).

Delegation has been described as the ability to assign work to a staff member. However, the most important element in delegation is the ability to assign to another the responsibility and authority to complete a task with the knowledge that the individual has the capability to

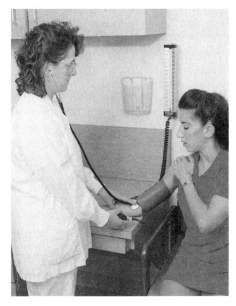

FIGURE 7–2. Unlicensed assistive personnel (UAP) may assist in many tasks, including measuring vital signs.

accomplish the task successfully. The judgment one uses in the act of delegation, not one's accountability for the act performed, is essentially the issue. All nurses, but especially the nurse manager, need to be aware of and trust the competencies of the staff members with whom they are working. The risk management of such a situation lies in whether the nurse making the assignment or delegating authority had reasonable knowledge that the delegatee had the competent ability to carry out the task. What better way to establish trust between team members than to have standardized protocols and competency levels that must be met by all staff members in particular job categories? These competencies should be extended to all staff who either float or are hired temporarily from registries to provide safe, competent care on fast-paced patient care units.

Delegation is the art of letting go and gaining the cooperation of others. Making assignments is easiest and most efficient if the components of delegation are followed. Effective delegation requires that (1) the task to be delegated is clearly identified; (2) patient needs are assessed; (3) the staff person is empowered to carry out activities to complete the task; and (4) a system of accountability is in place to monitor staff performance.

Identifying Tasks

Making assignments involves identifying and delegating specific tasks of the care of a patient to a staff person. The nurse manager assigns the care of several patients to each staff member. It is essential that the delegating nurse is aware of the care that each patient requires, and the strengths and weaknesses of the staff members assigned to the unit. Having information about the patients and the staff facilitates the nurse manager's ability to match skills, interests, and needs of both patients and staff. This matching process is essential to providing quality care and services to the patient and maximizing staff abilities and morale.

Assessing Need

An important method for assessing patient needs is walking rounds. Visit each patient daily. Observe how they function, both physically and cognitively, and any unusual problems they may have, such as a feeding tube or skin problem. Listen to what the patients have to say about the staff and about their needs. Answering a patient call light when all other staff members are busy is a great opportunity to observe a patient's abilities and demonstrates to the staff the manager's willingness to be part of the team. Another method for assessing patient need is to refer to the objective assessment measurement used by the facility or organization. Nursing homes utilize the minimum data set to assess patient needs, including their functional abilities and deficits. Such a standardized assessment form, or the care plan, can provide objective information for each patient on which to base assignments.

Some facilities or organizations use standardized acuity systems to facilitate making assignments. Acuity systems are standardized ways to measure each patient's needs, or the nursing tasks that need to be completed for each patient. They allow the nurse to compare patients in terms of the severity and acuity of their needs or the amount of nursing time that may be required to care for them. Most acuity systems measure aspects of patient care needs and group patients into categories based on these needs. Each category is typically assigned a name or value that corresponds to the amount of nursing time required to care for the average patient in that category. An example is an acuity system that categorizes patients as light, moderate, or heavy care. A patient in the light category may only need assistance with activities of daily living, whereas a patient in the heavy category may be totally dependent for all activities of daily living.

Acuity systems are used in making assignments by allocating patients by category to each staff member. The number of patients assigned to each staff member may depend on the patient and staff ratios (number of patients per each staff member) set by the organization or unit. If the acuity categories have numerical values, you may allocate a specific number of points to each staff person. If the facility uses an acuity system for facilitating staffing, be sure to ask for a thorough orientation on how the systems work and the basis on which the categories are determined.

Empowering Staff

Cooperation is necessary in delegation. The hands-on caregiver staff, who may be other LP/VNs or CNAs, are the experts in the nursing care of each of their patients. They need to be respected as such, involved in the planning of care, and empowered with the ability to make alterations in care (within their scope of practice and abilities) based on their assessment of the present needs of the patient. To empower the staff means that (1) their input in incorporated in the aspects of care that involve them; (2) information is shared with them regarding the care of the patient; (3) staffing models that empower should be used.

To provide the best care possible, staff must be well informed concerning changes in the patient and the plan of care. Verbal reports and walking rounds at the beginning and end of the shift help the staff and the nurse manager develop a frequent, regular system of communication and provide opportunities for input and feedback. Staff providing hands-on care need to have ready access to the formal, written plan of care and become accustomed to consulting it frequently.

Accountability

After the nurse manager becomes familiar with the needs of the patients and identifies a staffing model to make assignments, a system for holding staff accountable for the goals and responsibilities of their assignment is needed. Accountability requires that employees understand what is expected of them. In addition to the plan of care for each of their patients, do they know what other tasks and behaviors are expected? For example, when should they take breaks and where? Do they have other unit assignments such as ordering supplies or putting away supplies? How do they report changes in a patient's condition? These items may be reviewed in a unit orientation, but they may need review on a regular basis.

An accountability system requires some sort of reporting mechanism. This system may be verbal, written, or both. Documentation on flow sheets is a common system of accountability. These flow sheets provide written information that services were provided. They may also be used to document the outcome of these services from the staff perspective.

When nursing personnel are held accountable for their job responsibilities, it does not merely mean that the nurse manager corrects them when they do something wrong. It is equally important to commend staff when they meet or exceed expectations. Rewarding positive behaviors is often much more effective in improving performance than punishing behaviors.

Legal Considerations

Delegation is a very valuable tool; however, it has some unique, serious patient care and legal implications. Nurses practicing in the clinical setting must be concerned especially about the nursing tasks they delegate to unlicensed assistive personnel (Table 7–7). If care is improperly provided and harm results to the patient, the nurse will be held responsible. More and more frequently in malpractice lawsuits, licensed nurses are held liable for improper delegation or inadequate supervision of delegated tasks. Also, actions by state boards of nursing against a nurse's license based on delegation issues have been increasing.

TABLE 7–7
Avoiding Liability in Delegation

- Recognize when it happens.
- Review applicable state nurse practice act and regulations.
- Review applicable agency policies and procedures.
- Evaluate whether or not unlicensed assistive personnel may safely perform the task.
- Verify competency of the unlicensed person.
- Direct or supervise performance of the task.
- Assess the patient for the effectiveness of care performed.
- Ensure accurate documentation.
- Correct any situation when performance is inappropriate.

APPLYING LEADERSHIP AND MANAGEMENT

There is a subtle difference between leadership and management. Leadership focuses on people and inspires them to perform or change. Management focuses on getting the job done by planning, organizing, directing, and controlling people and activities. To be effective, managers must also have leadership abilities. Good nurses use many management and leadership skills in their varied professional roles.

Clinical Practice Roles

Nursing delivers its service to society through clinical practice roles. The teaching and administrative roles within the profession exist to support and represent the clinical practice roles. Circumstances, such as the availability of nurses, changing patient populations, changes in technology, hospital system variations, and altered financial conditions, lead to the development of new models of care delivery or variations in current models. Nurses use their knowledge of systems, the current circumstances, and the priorities of care to adjust the current model of care delivery or to create a new one.

Staff Nurse

The core role of nursing is the staff nurse role. Most nurses are staff nurses, and they deliver most of the nursing care directly to patients, whether in the hospital, long-term care, or home setting. He or she fulfills many functions in the delivery of patient care. These include care provider, decision-maker, patient advocate, team member, communicator, and educator.

Whether working in a hospital, clinic, or office setting, or in the community, the staff nurse initiates the nursing process. He or she assesses the patient and family, determines nursing diagnoses, establishes a plan of care (nursing orders), and evaluates the outcome of the care. In addition, the staff nurse consults with other health care professionals, reports the most current patient status, and coordinates the care by these professionals. The staff nurse uses management skills to integrate the nursing care plan with the therapy plans of the other health care professionals and leadership skills to coordinate the interdisciplinary care for the patient.

Beginning Managers

Gradually, staff nurses gain experience managing care for patients, and assisting team members. Eventually, they also serve as a resource for new nurses. These enhanced activities are an indication to supervisors that staff nurses are ready to assume beginning management functions. Two examples of this early management role are team leader and charge nurse.

The team leader directs the actions of a group of nurses and ensures quality of care delivery. The charge nurse is responsible for a nursing unit for a particular shift. He or she makes management decisions and supervises the unit as needed to provide quality patient care on that shift. The charge nurse and team leader are typically resources for other staff members and may be pulled into issues that require interdepartmental or interdisciplinary problem solving.

Unit Management

Permanent management roles at the hospital unit level are typically the head nurse and assistant head nurse. The head nurse role is a pivotal role within the hospital. In many organizations, he or she is recognized as a department head and is held accountable for the 24-hour operation of the nursing unit. Operations include such functions as staff scheduling and supervision, budget management, staff education, and quality patient care. The head nurse also provides a vital communication link among patients, direct caregivers, and the administration. Responsibilities include alerting the administration to changing patient needs and care preferences as well as changing staff characteristics. The head nurse will represent the administration to the staff and patients and communicate changes in the organization that may affect them.

The assistant head nurse provides support and aid to the head nurse. He or she performs functions delegated by the head nurse (e.g., hiring, evaluating, and counseling staff; preparing work schedules; and preparing and monitoring the unit budget). Additionally, the assistant head nurse often serves as a unit-based clinical resource and educator.

Middle Managers

Depending on the size and complexity of the hospital or agency, there may be several levels of middle management. Between the head nurse or coordinator there may be managers with titles of supervisor, assistant director, associate director, or assistant administrator. These middle managers are usually responsible for the activities of several departments and programs. They spend more time in strategic planning and interdepartmental problem solving than the head nurse, but spend less of their time dealing with day-to-day patient care management than the head nurse does.

Upper Level Management

The nurse executive has a variety of titles and duties, depending on the type and complexity of the institution or health care agency. Some of the titles are vice president, associate administrator, or director of nursing. The nurse executive is an administrator and a leader of professionals. Because he or she is involved in strategic planning and decision making for the institution, the nurse executive must effectively negotiate with nonclinical administrators and the medical director (the other top-level clinical administrator). The nurse executive also must be able to lead, influence, and represent nursing professionals.

To be effective in all of these management roles, people must be skilled in the techniques of planning, organizing, directing, and controlling. The proportion of time spent doing each of these activities varies with each role. The beginning managers, head nurse, and assistant head nurse primarily focus on current operations and patient care management. The nurse executive primarily focuses on strategic planning and issues within the agency that affect nursing practice or issues with the community or other agencies. A manager's success depends on strong management techniques and effective leadership practices. The higher the level of the manager, the more essential it is for him or her to be an effective leader. Nurse executives are expected to be leaders within their agency and in the nursing profession itself. Effective nurse executives establish circumstances that allow nurses to function as professionals when providing quality patient care.

Managing Change

Change can be defined as growth or learning experience. Managers must be masters of the change process. They need to be able to assess a situation and anticipate future needs, to determine when change is needed, and to implement the needed change. Managers also must be able to manage change that is imposed by others.

Managers need to know how to overcome resistance to change in themselves, their staff, and the overall organization. Lack of knowledge, inaccurate information, fear of the unknown, threats to status or position, and threats to economic benefits can cause resistance to change. Education and enhanced communication are the best ways to reduce resistance caused by a lack of information or inaccurate information. Participation and involvement are effective approaches when the initiators of the change do not have all the information they need to design the change and when others have the power to resist the change. When people are resisting the change because of emotional adjustment problems, the best interventions are facilitation and support. Negotiation and agreement may be appropriate when the change adversely affects the person's position or economic status.

People can control their perceptions and reactions to change by being aware of emotional reactions associated with change and by actively seeking information, increasing communication, and getting involved in the change process. Those who perceive change as an opportunity for learning and personal growth see it as positive and offer less resistance to change.

To implement change effectively, nurse managers must assess the implications of any change for themselves and their staff and must intervene by providing needed communication, information, support, and involvement. For instance, illness represents a change for patients and their family members. The nurse increases communication, teaches, involves the patient and family in care, and offers support to ease patient and family adjustment to illness.

UTILIZING POWER EFFECTIVELY

Being new to management, the nurse manager needs to understand power and how to use it effectively. The culture of an organization may be very subtle, but either through observation of formal structures (e.g., the organizational chart) or informal structures, the new manager should try to identify where the power is located and learn how to access that power to get a job done.

Just as important as gaining and developing power is the ability to do what is right with power, not only to use it for personal gain. The concept of power includes action, knowledge, position, judgment, and perception. Power is not static, it is not a place. Power is intoxicating and its results can be devastating to staff and an organization if used in a nonproductive manner. It needs to be activated for the good of the group.

A new manager has the power that is associated with the hierarchy of position. However, that power may be eroded if not used effectively or if allowed to be usurped by another. Power becomes another tool for the manager to manage a department effectively. Even though it may appear superficial, it is important for nurse managers to look the part in order to receive the respect that is due them. Dress as a professional nurse manager, act as a professional nurse manager—body language and communication styles exude power. That is not to say that aggressive behavior denotes power. Knowing when to use which behavioral style (e.g., aggressiveness, assertiveness, passivity, submission) is an important element of gaining a power base.

Power should never be used to dominate or totally control staff. Respect the individuality, responsibility, and creativity of staff and use power to develop and mentor them to be more involved in team efforts. Delegate, mentor, and manage through performance goals and expectations. Leadership is intertwined with effective use of power.

Just as important as communicating power to staff is the need to gain influence with superiors. An old management saying goes, "the job of a manager is to make his/her boss look good." The purpose of a nursing middle management position is to manage a patient care department, meeting quality, regulatory/accreditation, and financial objectives. The senior manager is responsible for a number of departments, overseeing the strategic direction and leadership. A good manager is aware of the familial relationship and nurtures positive growth of that important relationship with a supervisor.

Power develops and is recognized in a variety of ways. It is important to understand the different types of power so one can identify it in oneself and others. Power types are also referred to as bases of power or the source from which the power comes.

Expert Power

Expert power is the strongest power base for nursing. The need is for an expert nurse to be there to mentor, support, and teach the novice nurse. If a new nurse is in trouble with a patient and wants another nursing opinion as to how to manage the situation, he or she usually will seek out an older, more experienced nurse.

Being an expert is powerful. It also is a positive, nonaggressive way to have power. Managers with power based on expert knowledge do not have to engage in power struggles or other types of power battles because when one is an expert, that is an obvious fact that is not questioned. Power based on expertise does not have to be advertised or listed as an agenda item at meetings. It is a fact that others know because of the expert work of the person with that type of power. It is always noticed. Experts in a work area can be identified easily, because they simply are the expert and their power is noted by others.

Not everyone will be an expert at every aspect of the profession. It is important to determine an area of interest and become proficient at it. The area could be administering medications, giving pressure ulcer treatments, making schedules with the right mix of people, or effectively managing groups of employees or patients. Expert power is the strongest power base; therefore, it is one that should be recognized, respected, and developed.

Reward Power

Reward power derives from an interesting power base. The person with this type of power has the ability to give rewards to others. This is like allowing a child to go to the movies with a friend if the household chores assigned the child are completed. The parent has power over the rewards given a minor child.

Nurse managers also have a strong power base if their manager has given it to them. A middle manager is responsible for the schedule and with that who gets weekends and holidays off duty. The manager has power over vacation leave and salary increases as well, and is the person responsible for the employee's evaluation. This is a strong power base.

Compare the reward power base with the expert power base. What differences are there? The person with an expert power base generally does not or cannot use it to manipulate other employees. It is possible, however, for the person with reward power to do just that to others. Not everyone who has a reward power base uses it to manipulate people, but it is possible and does happen on occasion. The concept of giving and receiving rewards often alters a person's behavior. The manager may identify and reward favorites or "pets" with the preferred schedules. This type of power can lead to what is referred to as "brownnosing" behavior from employees. Reward power is quickly recognized when people are being manipulated because conditions in the work environment are unfair. People complain about it and the possibility for conflict is high.

Remember that not all reward power-based managers use their positions to manipulate others. Many are fair and committed, giving rewards to those who have earned them while using the possibility of a reward to motivate someone else to change behaviors that are undesirable. Is is important for those who possess reward power to use the rewards carefully and with fairness as a mechanism to support the work of the team's responsibilities.

Coercive Power

The coercion power base is exactly what the manipulative use of reward power turns into, coercion. It occurs when someone has reward power and uses it specifically to negatively treat employees. The focus of coercive power is not to assist others to improve or contribute more to the work team but instead to specifically hurt and punish others. This manager has reward power, but chooses to use it in a negative manner.

A nurse manager who has coercive power may give a formal reprimand when a quiet teaching moment would have been more effective; may assign undesirable jobs to a nurse who is showing creativity and initiative at work; or may hold the threat of being fired over people who question the manager's thinking. This is an unhealthy power base and must be avoided by nurse managers who wish to be successful.

Legitimate Power

Legitimate power indicates that the person has earned the power that actually accompanies a job and its responsibilities.

The nurse with the title of nurse manager, head nurse, team leader, charge nurse, or others that are similar has major responsibilities and the power to do the job required. The power is based on the authority that someone higher in the power chain has given to the nurse manager and the nurse's position in the hierarchy of the organization.

Referent Power

Referent power is a nice, caring-type of power that many people use, but do not recognize as a formal power base. It develops from feelings of admiration and respect for another person. For example, if a nurse knew a significant nurse leader, and shared his or her views from a personal conversation with him or her while attending an educational workshop on nursing as a profession, he or she would quickly develop referent power. People would respect the nurse because he or she had a relationship with such a significant person.

Sometimes people want advice on personal or professional matters. Generally, they seek out someone they admire or have referent power toward, but don't recognize it as such. Referent power people often-times do not recognize that they have it. They are the type of people who work in a focused manner to do things right. They usually are successful in their personal and professional lives and emanate self-confidence and integrity. These people have power because of the way they live their lives and their willingness to share their lives with others.

KEY POINTS

- Nurses are professionals responsible for providing a service through effective leadership behaviors and management skills.
- Leadership is the ability to influence others to strive for a goal or vision or to change. Management is getting the job done or the goal accomplished through planning, organizing, directing, and controlling.
- The management process is similar to the problem-solving and the nursing processes because all are based on the scientific or research process.
- As managers, nurses need to be skilled in problem solving, communicating, and managing change.
- The five steps of the problem-solving process are identifying and analyzing the problem, determining possible solutions, consider-ing the consequences of each possible solution and choosing a solution, implementing the solution, and evaluating the results.
- Change is inevitable. People can influence their own perceptions and reactions to change by being aware of the emotions associated within and by actively seeking information, increasing communi-cation, and getting involved in the change process.
- New nursing graduates have many options available in work settings and roles within nursing.

CRITICAL THINKING ACTIVITIES

1. Compare and contrast the advantages of team nursing with pri-mary nursing for the patient. Do the same for the nurses in the two situations.
2. Considering your skill and knowledge, select the model in which you would like to participate. List your reasons.
3. If you were practicing under case management, analyze how you would collaborate with other nurses and with other staff members.

CASE STUDY

When power is used to promote oneself or one's ideas without regard for the larger group, it is being used for negative purposes. Consider the situation where a group of health care providers is working together on a hospital unit and a new middle manager is hired. This manager comes from another hospital in the city where he managed an efficient unit but left because of disagreements with the administrator. After one month on the unit, the manager decides, without using good change theory, that everyone has to work full time and the unit must change back to 8-hour shifts. He makes it clear that those who cannot make the change may have an opportunity to apply for positions in other areas of the hospital. The manager has the support of administration because of a desire that administration has to empower managers, and there is no apparent recourse to the problem. Within one more month, several of the experienced, part-time nurses had left the unit, and others who were in school, because the 12-hour shifts allowed them to do that and work, had either dropped out of school or left the unit. The manager has not had any trouble filling the vacant positions by hiring former employees from his previous job. He frequently says he can't work 12-hour shifts because of his pets.

Case Discussion

What type of reaction do you have to this scenario? Discuss the importance of meeting the needs of the larger group. This negative use of power allowed the manager to surround himself with nurses he already knew, as opposed to nurses who knew the unit. What assessments might have been completed before the changes were made? Discuss the possible ways nurses could approach a manager if presented with such a situation. Would assertive communication focused on group needs be appropriate? Could the number of people on the work team be used as a source of power?

Topics for Nursing Inquiry

- What are the leadership behaviors of staff nurses who are identified as experts by their peers?
- What are the relative priorities of various management skills of staff nurses at different career stages?
- What is the impact of varying leadership styles of head nurses on staff nurse job satisfaction and retention?
- What effect do various staff nurse roles and the use of assistive personnel have on patient care outcomes?

CASE STUDY

You are an LPN/LVN recently assigned to work on the skilled nursing unit of an acute care hospital. You are responsible for a team of five nursing assistants. One of the NAs has worked in long-term care for many years. She is a caring employee and does a good job, but does not have a restorative approach. She would rather do for her patients than encourage them to do for themselves. You notice that she does not walk her residents and frequently applies vest restraints to keep the patients "safe."

1. Because you are new and are not sure why the NA is behaving in this manner, you realize the need to gather more information. You set up a counseling interview with the employee. What should you discuss at this meeting?
   During the counseling session, the NA informs you that she does not feel old people should be made to walk. She just wants to keep them clean, safe, and happy. She understands your expectations to help the residents regain function, but is fearful to allow them to be unrestrained. She agrees to spend more time in the therapy department, which you arrange, to learn more about restorative care. After a week you notice that her patients still are not being walked and most remain in vest restraints during the day. When you ask, she says that there was not time to go to the therapy department as you arranged.
2. What is your next step in helping this employee to improve her performance?
   This strategy is ineffective in changing the NA's behavior. She is still not using a restorative approach with the patients. In addition, several other areas of her performance are not up to standards. You see the need to develop a performance improvement plan.
3. What do you include in the performance improvement plan for this individual NA?

Case Study Suggestions

1. You ask the NA to see you when she has a few moments available and schedule a time to meet that is convenient for both of you. Meet in privacy, either in an office or in an area where other staff cannot overhear. Discuss the behaviors that you wish changed. You want the patients to be assisted to walk or at least stand every day. You want them to have active or passive range of motion each

day and you want the NA to use the wedge cushion or other restraint alternatives identified in each patient's plan of care, instead of the vest restraints. Ask the NA why she has not been providing this restorative care. Identify what can be done to help the NA correct her behavior and begin providing restorative care.

2. Another private interview with the employee is in order. Discuss reasons for the employee's resistance and try to problem solve to remove those reasons. Give the NA positive reinforcement for the tasks done well, but emphasize that the skills in restorative care need to improve for her overall performance to be acceptable. Be specific about the behaviors you want the NA to demonstrate. Inform the NA that you plan to arrange a specific date and time for her to visit the therapy department. You also arrange coverage for the NA's patients on the unit. Ask the NA if there is anything else you can do to help her improve. Let the NA know that you consider this discussion a verbal warning and that her behavior needs to change. If it does not change, progressive discipline should follow.

3. You complete a performance review on the NA and specifically identify the performance standards that she is not meeting. You meet with the employee to discuss the review and identify behaviors that need to be changed, including the need to focus on restorative care. You let the NA know that although this is not the usual time for a review, she has areas where she is particularly strong and other areas where she needs to improve. The performance review and the compilation of a performance improvement plan give the NA specific ideas on what needs to be done. Together you discuss what should be included in the plan:

   a. Determine the performance standards the NA needs to meet and specific goals for her behaviors.
   b. Set a time frame for achievement. Because you have been talking with the NA about restorative care over the last few weeks, the time frame for achievement of this goal may be shorter than the rest. Set up the next meeting when you can discuss progress with the NA.
   c. Determine what you can do to help the NA achieve the goals.
   d. Outline the consequences if the NA does not meet the goals. Be sure to discuss the potential consequences with your supervisor before you include them in the performance plan. Consequences may range from termination to progressive discipline to transfer off the unit.

BIBLIOGRAPHY

Barnum, B. S. (1994). Realities in nursing practice: A strategic view. *Nursing & Health Care, 15*(8), 400–405.

Bellman, G. M. (1992). *Getting things done when you are not in charge.* New York: Fireside.

Catalano, J. T. (1996). *Contemporary professional nursing.* Philadelphia: Davis.

Covey, S. R. (1991). Principle-centered leadership. In S. R. Covey, *The 7 Habits of Highly Effective People* (pp. 40–47, 138). New York: Summit.

Douglass, L. M. (1992). *The effective nurse leader and manager* (4th ed). St. Louis: C. V. Mosby.

Dunhamp-Taylor, J., Fisher, E., & Kinion, E. (1993). Experiences, events, people: Do they influence the leadership style of nurse executives? *Journal of Nursing Administration, 23*(7/8), 30–34.

Gillies, D. A. (1994). *Nursing management: A systems approach* (3rd ed.). Philadelphia: W. B. Saunders.

Gunden, E., & Crissman, S. (1992). Leadership skills for empowerment. *Nursing Administration Quarterly, 16*(3), 6–10.

Hitt, W. D. (1990). *Ethics and leadership: Putting theory into practice.* Columbus: Battelle.

Kerfoot, K. M. (1994). Leaders: Yesterday, today, and tomorrow. In R. Spitzer-Lehmann (Ed.), *Nursing management desk reference: Concepts, skills, and strategies.* Philadelphia: W. B. Saunders.

Kouzes, J. M., & Posner, B. Z. (1993). *Credibility.* San Francisco: Jossey-Bass.

Mark, B. A. (1994). The emerging role of the nurse manager: Implications for educational preparation. *Journal of Nursing Administration, 24*(1), 48–55.

Marquis, B. L., & Huston, C. J. (1996). *Leadership roles and management functions in nursing theory and application* (2nd ed.). Philadelphia: Lippincott-Raven.

Marriner-Torrey, A. (1992). *Guide to nursing management* (8th ed.). St. Louis: C. V. Mosby.

Parker, Y. (1996). *Damn good resume guide: A crash course in resume writing.* Berkeley, CA: Ten Speed Press.

Wilkinson, A. P. (1998, June). Nursing malpractice. *Nursing Today 98, 28*(6), 34–38.

Leadership and Management in Nursing   **257**

INTERNET RESOURCES

Agency for Healthcare Policy & Research
http://www.ahcpr.gov
Department of Health and Human Services
http://www.os.dhhs.gov
Health Care Financing Administration
http://www.hcfa.gov
Health on the Net
http://www.hon.ch
Hospital Web
http://neuro-www.mgh.harvard.edu/hospitalweb.shtml
National Institutes of Health
http://www.nih.gov
United Nations
http://www.un.gov

CHAPTER 8

Career Management

OVERVIEW

Nursing is an exciting and challenging career, but the transition from student to practicing nurse is not easy—even after coursework is completed. This chapter provides information on issues of concern to those serious about a career in nursing. Subjects discussed include role transition from student to graduate, employer expectations, self-assessment, goal setting, the relevance of the political process for nurses, recruitment, the application process, the post-interview process, malpractice insurance, N-CLEX preparation, and self-care strategies.

OBJECTIVES

Upon completion of this chapter, the reader should be able to:

- Develop a list of personal career goals.
- Identify at least six expectations employers have of new graduates.
- Create a professional résumé, a sample letter of application.
- Identify strategies that assist in the transition from student to graduate.
- Develop a plan for maintaining personal competency in nursing.

⟫ **KEY TERMS**

Cover letter	Reality shock
Mentor	Résumé
Networking	

INTRODUCTION

Nursing is one of the most rewarding professions, and it can also be one of the most frustrating. Nurses seldom find their specific situation in nursing exactly as they thought it would be. This process of "reality shock" is not confined to nursing, however. It is described in many professions as the graduate moves from the world of academics to the world of work and begins to adjust to new demands and expectations.

The work environment is demanding to the new graduate. This transition does not need to be difficult though. The search for employment should be managed as any other assignment. Homework will be necessary. Sufficient knowledge of personal needs, strengths, and areas of growth assists job hunters in the process. There are many new challenges and new responsibilities, and planning ahead will assist in making a successful transition. Being prepared and knowing what to expect will help in maintaining a positive, healthy attitude.

ROLE TRANSITION AND REALITY SHOCK

When a new graduate from any educational experience enters the workforce, he or she experiences a major change. Nursing is no different (and in some respects it is worse). There is a difference between theoretical learning and clinical practice. The information learned in school is referred to as "knowing that" information. It is a knowledge foundation base for practicing nursing.

There is a second type of knowledge that is necessary to move from a novice to an expert nurse. This is the "knowing how" information. This is the material that nurses learn while practicing their art in the real world of nursing. Developing knowing how knowledge comes from caring for a patient or a category of patients over time and learning, for example, that a small piece of candy is better for a particular individual's hypoglycemic reaction than orange juice. This information evolves without explanation while the nurse is performing the day-to-day responsibilities of the profession. Often it cannot be explained. For example, although many, if not most, adults know how to ride a bicycle or swim, few can explain how to do it. The bike rider may receive a great deal of knowing that knowledge, but still cannot ride until he or she gets on the bike and does it. Some nursing experts refer to this as intuitive knowing, which is based on the solid foundation of theoretical or knowing that knowledge.

The actual practice of nursing requires extensive knowing that knowledge, and that is the purpose of school; however, after graduation the nurse proceeds to the knowing how part of his or her education. Challenges are to be expected because not everyone follows the textbook procedures so carefully learned in school; not everyone understands how he or she knows something, but instead urges the new graduate to believe and trust in his or her knowledge; not every nurse is an expert nurse.

The new graduate may encounter high and unrealistic expectations combined with an inability to effect positive change. Realistically, all too often one's focus is directed toward getting the essentials of the job done in the shift time allowed. The new graduate may feel that it is impossible to administer the quality of nursing care needed within the limitations of the current health care system. All of this describes what our nursing educators and experts call **reality shock**.

Nurses have reacted to reality shock in a variety of ways, including leaving nursing altogether, returning to school for answers to an imperfect problem, or going from one job to another, looking for "greener pastures." Some nurses have difficulty balancing what they were taught and what the real world demands of them. Many lack the personal strength to practice based on correctness and principles they know are correct. It sometimes seems easier to "go along with the group." The challenge for the nurse is to develop the ability to work with a wide variety of professionals and paraprofessionals to promote the health and wellness of all people in his or her care while at the same time developing their own nursing expertise.

The perfect solution does not yet exist to combat the far-reaching effects of reality shock. However, a discussion of goal setting provides the basis to review nursing strengths and to identify those skill areas requiring study and refinement.

NURSE PRACTICE ACT

A nurse practice act is the law of each state that defines nursing and what the various levels of nurses may legally do in their practice. The act differs from state to state; some are specific and some are general. It is essential that new nurses assume the responsibility to thoroughly understand the licensed nurse's scope of practice in the state where they work. Most often the wording of a nurse practice act is purposefully general to allow for changes and growth in the organization without enacting new legislation for each change. In a general sense, the scope of practice for a Licensed Practical/Vocational Nurse (LP/VN) focuses on the health needs of patients in hospitals, residents in nursing homes, and members of the community. It often is required that the LP/VN work under the supervision of a registered nurse (RN) or physician.

The policies and procedures of all employers should follow the nurse practice act. If they do not, it is the nurse's responsibility to know the law and follow it in spite of the hospital's policies. If a nurse does not follow the law as outlined, he or she may be in violation and his or her license could be in jeopardy.

SELF-ASSESSMENT AND GOAL SETTING

Each nurse is his or her own best evaluator. This is because no one knows more about that person and his or her abilities than he or she does. Self-evaluation means examining one's assets as well as one's defects, or areas requiring growth. Two points that should always be included are self-sufficiency and self-confidence. The rule of success is "have a positive attitude and know yourself."

It is impossible for the new graduate nurse to function well in every area. Individual likes and dislikes influence performance. Seeking assistance and collaboration from those who want to help is an excellent self-evaluation strategy. Nurses should accept criticism gracefully and try to profit from it. It is not always necessary to agree, but it is important to be realistic and honest. A careful study of one's personality, abilities, and achievements in nursing helps people decide the area of nursing for which they are best suited.

A good exercise is to establish a career plan. What are realistic goals for next year, three years from now, and even five years? This may involve delaying plans for advancement so a better groundwork of additional education may be laid. Perhaps it means a rigorous schedule

ASK YOURSELF

What Is Your Career Plan?

Determine how your competencies and abilities correspond to your expectations as well as to those of potential employers. Career goals need to be both short and long term. This means that goals are not static; they must be realistic, personal, and flexible. Although both long-term and short-term goals will be revised as your life evolves, they will guide you in making day-to-day decisions more effectively. Be ready to consider alternative goals and a variety of pathways to one goal.

of continuing education courses to obtain a certificate in a specialized nursing area. All types of career plans need and deserve advance planning.

Mentoring

It is not uncommon to hear nurses on all levels complain about the lack of support they receive as they try to master a new role. Novice nurses often feel overwhelmed, but they usually learn and master the profession much faster if they have someone to guide and advise them through their transition. This person is known as a mentor. A **mentor** is a more skilled or more experienced person who serves as a role model, teaches, sponsors, encourages, counsels, and befriends a less skilled or less experienced person for the purpose of promoting the latter's professional and/or personal development. Mentoring functions are carried out within the context of an ongoing, caring relationship between the mentor and the novice.

Mentoring is done in many ways, including counseling, role modeling, and teaching. It is a behavior that is soundly grounded in the theory of caring. Nurses need to demonstrate caring behaviors for themselves, each other, and patients. Unfortunately, most nurses are lucky if they have one or two mentors throughout their career. The reality is that there are few committed mentors in nursing.

The challenge for a new graduate is to find one. The benefits are of a tremendous value. Every new job has a great deal of new information and skills to master, and a mentor is the perfect person to assist in that mastery.

TABLE 8–1
Criteria for Choosing a Mentor

- Has an interest in the same clinical practice you are interested in learning
- Demonstrates a high level of skill in your area of interest
- Is receptive to questions from you and others
- Integrates teaching into the questions being answered or explanations being made

To identify a mentor is the first challenge. The new nurse should look around and locate someone who demonstrates the behaviors that he or she wants to achieve. It is necessary to evaluate the person as to being receptive to mentoring and their willingness to explain and clarify information as needed (Table 8–1).

Most people are honored to be asked to mentor someone in the nuances of nursing. Some react with surprise, and others may express concern over their abilities. Others may even discredit themselves and state that they do not have the ability. The new nurse should be clear in what he or she wants and ask in a pleasant and nondemanding manner. Most professionals are aware of the need to mentor the less experienced people on a health care team. It is just good business; however, they may not know how to go about mentoring because they have not seen many role models for this behavior.

There is a danger associated with mentoring. There are individuals who are toxic mentors. This term describes four types of mentors who are destructive. The four types are avoiders, dumpers, blockers, and destroyers. They do not assist new nurses with career growth and the transition from student to nurse. The nursing profession needs to find ways to deal with these negative behaviors to minimize their impact. The novice nurse needs to recognize the characteristics and avoid people who demonstrate them.

The "avoiders" are nonresponsive people who are unavailable or inaccessible. If an issue is brought to them, they generally do not follow up. The "dumpers," by contrast, throw people into a new role or position and let them fail. They function on the "sink or swim" motto that produces a great deal of transition trauma. "Blockers" refuse to help, withhold information needed to succeed, or stifle the development of the individual by hovering too closely. Finally, "destroyers" tear down an individual by undermining in subtle or overt ways to destroy the

Table 8–2

Five Self-Mentoring Strategies

- Interact with people. Ask questions, listen, and clarify what you know with others to enhance your understanding.
- Find and use references. Read books and journal articles.
- Observe people who are knowledgeable and who have insight.
- Enroll in educational programs, especially ones that include skill practice.
- Figure out solutions for yourself; reflect on them; and work them through on your own.

novice nurse's confidence. They criticize without regard for the quality of work.

Sometimes there is not a person available. In that situation a new nurse needs to recognize that he or she still needs mentoring. Using the self-mentoring techniques described in Table 8–2 will assist him or her with role transition.

Networking

One of the strategies to a smooth transition and continued professional success is **networking**. Like mentoring, networking is a skill that is not fully recognized or adopted by the nursing profession. It is, however, an effective method for informing people about personal goals, concerns, or desires in an informal manner.

A well-networked mentor is a real bonus. A well-networked mentor will pass along news about conferences, job openings, and items of concern in your clinical practice.

How can a soon-to-be graduate start networking? He or she may get started in several ways. One way is to start with local nursing instructors. They know about jobs and application strategies and also have an objective view of a student's strengths and areas of needed improvement. The best strategy is to make an appointment with the instructor. By making the appointment, the student will act like a professional and impress the faculty member. During the meeting, the student nurse should explain his or her goals and ask the questions that need to be answered.

The idea of making an appointment with an instructor fits into the development of a good network base. Nurses often can increase their power and influence, both personally and professionally, by forming alliances with other groups and individuals. The alliance provides a mechanism for sharing of information, clarifying information, and making decisions. By being well networked, a person has "the edge" in terms of additional information and opinions of people with more experience or facts. It is impossible to know ahead of time which networking contact will provide the best reward. That is why nurses should form several alliances. Most nurses plan on working for extended periods of time, and most nursing careers are not short-term experiences. A nursing career can be rich in experiences with others, information, and opportunity if a network of contacts is developed and nurtured.

Commitment to Lifelong Learning

A final strategy for successful entry into the nursing profession is commitment to lifelong learning. It is a concept that is important to success in any licensed position. Commitment to lifelong learning does not mean that an RN licensure, a master's degree, or a Ph.D. is needed. Rather, it means avoiding stagnation—allowing the information learned in nursing school to become stale.

Going back to school for an additional license or a degree in nursing is one option. Also valuable is conscientious attention to conferences and workshops to keep on the cutting edge of nursing practice. Nurses cannot afford to maintain a job without pursuing a learning program. The obvious detriments are the danger to patients and the possibility of malpractice. Neither the nurse nor the patient is safe if the nurse's knowledge is outdated.

One way to enhance both networking ability and lifelong learning goals is to belong to a professional organization such as the National Federation of Licensed Practical Nurses (NFLPN). This is an experience that allows LP/VNs to know other LP/VN leaders in their state and throughout the nation. One of the main purposes of this organization is to sponsor continuing education programs. It is an organization that provides nurses with a mechanism for meeting some of their goals.

Continuing Education

Every nurse has an obligation to society to maintain competence and continue practicing high-quality, safe care. Continuing education may occur through learning on the job, through reading of professional publications, or through attending classes. There are television courses, programmed instruction programs, and examinations related to journal articles.

In-Service Education. Many hospitals, as well as other places of employment, have in-service education programs. When a nurse secures a new position, the first in-service education that he or she receives is a program of orientation. If specific procedures must be performed, a series of concentrated classes may follow. An example of an institution using orientation in-service education is a rehabilitation hospital. Although the licensed nurse may already be familiar with range of motion exercises, these and other pertinent procedures are reviewed with new personnel.

Each hospital also has its own definite nursing care procedures, and personnel are required to follow these techniques rather than those previously learned. This uniformity helps ensure safety to patients and personnel. Some institutions provide follow-up classes to keep their employees abreast of current trends in patient care. Other in-service educational programs include special classes in the administration of medicines, operating room techniques, labor and delivery care, and cardiopulmonary resuscitation.

These classes are given on duty time. Because they are offered for the advancement of the employee, nurses should take advantage of them. No one should ever need to be forced to attend these classes. Financially, it is costly to the institution to offer such programs, but the advances made in nursing care as a result compensate for this cost.

Conventions and Workshops. Conventions and workshops are held locally, statewide, regionally, and nationally in a variety of forms. They may be offered or sponsored by alumni organizations, state organizations, and professional organizations. In addition, one- to three-day workshops are frequently offered. No one can expect to attend every convention offered; however, many hospitals make provisions for their employees to attend some educational conventions and workshops. Other nurses will request days off or request vacation days to attend professional association conventions and workshops. Programs offered on a local level are usually of shorter duration, and attendance presents fewer problems. Every day new advances, techniques, and methods of nursing care are being developed. Unless nurses become familiar with these developments and adopt them according to the policies of the hospital or institution, they gradually become less efficient, and their activities are limited.

Professional Journals and Publications. Reading articles from professional journals is valuable. Some journals are published especially for the licensed practical/vocational nurse. These include the Journal of Practical Nursing, Journal of Nursing Care, and other state and local publications.

The *Journal of Practical Nursing* is published by the National Association for Practical Nurse Education and Service. It is a monthly publication that keeps the nurse informed about national activities in the practical/vocational nursing group. It contains articles on nursing topics, upcoming events, available positions, new books and pamphlets, and activities occurring in various states.

The *Journal of Nursing Care* is published by Health Science Division, Technomic Publishing Company. It is a monthly publication that contains information about and activities of the National Federation of Licensed Practical Nurses. It includes reports from committees representing practical/vocational nursing, progress of practical/vocational nursing education programs, and any announcements the national headquarters desires to convey to its state or local members.

Nurses should become familiar with state and local publications. They are usually in the form of bulletins, journals, or magazines. They contain valuable information concerning the officers of the state and local divisions of professional organizations, plus events, programs, achievements, and happenings in the local vicinity.

Because procedures and techniques may change with new developments in medicine, maintaining proficiency by periodically reading new texts and references by leading publishers in nursing is essential for the licensed nurse. New publications are also advertised in most professional journals.

Post-licensure Programs. Post-licensure programs may be very beneficial to a licensed practical/vocational nurse who does not feel adequately prepared to assume responsibilities in a particular field. Some instructors and administrative personnel believe that it is wise for a new nurse to work for six months to one year in a general hospital to gain necessary experience. During student days some practical experience is acquired, but theory is emphasized. After graduation, limited theoretical knowledge is gained, and emphasis is placed on practical experience. After a year spent in a general hospital, the licensed practical/vocational nurse has sufficient background to specialize in one particular area and is equipped with a varied background sufficient for functioning smoothly and efficiently. Before enrolling in a post-licensure program, a nurse should investigate to see if it is an accredited program. Consideration must be given to all factors of time, cost, and living expenses needed. Some programs may mean living away from home or even in another state.

The post-licensure programs available may be found in monthly publications from local, state, or national organizations. They list the courses offered, the dates, and the locations where they are offered.

Refresher Courses. Refresher courses are offered by nursing schools, local organizations, or state and national organizations. They are offered to those wishing to bring themselves up to date with current trends in nursing care. The length of the course may vary with individual groups, material being taught, and different instructors. Many schools of practical/vocational nursing are now offering courses to their alumni and other interested licensed practical/vocational nurses. The most commonly offered course is administration of medications.

Local branches of the American National Red Cross offer courses such as first aid, cardiopulmonary resuscitation, swimming, and water safety. The procedures taught in these courses are current and serve as valuable aids to nursing and non-nursing persons. Television and computers are being used today to give educational courses in useful subjects for continuing education. Many of these programs award certificates on completion of the course, or the course credits may be applied to a continuing degree or certificate program. Notices of these programs may be found in the daily newspaper, the Internet, television guides, through local hospital education departments, and health care agencies. These notices are often posted on library bulletin boards or announced at various professional meetings.

COMPETENCIES AND EMPLOYERS' EXPECTATIONS

Another aspect of securing the perfect job is to be clear about what is expected of new nurses. In general all employers have the right to expect an employee to be well educated for the position being applied for and to have the skills and knowledge that represent that level of education, licensure, and experience.

Employers often ask for further clarification of competence. Have these graduates only the necessary theoretical knowledge regarding the skill? Have they actually performed the skill? If so, was it in a practice laboratory only, or was it in a patient care situation? Does competence mean that the new graduate can function independently, or will some supervision still be needed?

What is expected of the new graduate varies in different health care agencies and in different geographical areas. Expectations are affected by various factors in the community, such as whether there are nursing programs in that community and whether new graduates come from one or from many different schools. The acuity of the patient care load and the types of services offered by an agency may also affect expectations. The Joint Commission on the Accreditation of Healthcare Organizations (JCAHO) has a criterion requiring that accredited institutions monitor and ensure the competence of their staff. This requires that an institution identify expected competencies for staff and then design an assessment method. As institutions move to comply with this standard, most are directing their initial efforts toward technical skills, because these are more easily identified and assessed. The basic competencies that employers expect of newly graduated licensed nurses are discussed below.

Possess the necessary theoretical background for safe patient care and for decision making. Many employers believe that new graduates today are competent in this area. For example, the new nurse should understand the signs and symptoms of an insulin reaction, recognize it when it occurs, and know what nursing actions should be taken. The new nurse must know when an emergency or complication is occurring and secure medical help for the patient when that is needed.

Use the nursing process in a systematic way. This includes gathering information for assessment, planning, intervention, and evaluation. New graduates should be able to participate in the development of plans of care as well as follow plans such as care pathways that have been developed in that agency.

Recognize own abilities and limitations. To provide safe care, the nurse must identify when a situation requires greater expertise or knowledge and when assistance is needed. Employers may be able to assist if nurses ask for help and direction, but cannot accept the risk to patients created by nurses who do not know their own limitations.

Use communication skills effectively with patients and coworkers. In every setting there are patients and families who are anxious, depressed, suffering loss, or experiencing other types of emotional distress. The nurse is expected to respond appropriately to these individuals and to facilitate their coping and adaptation. Effective communication skills are essential to the functioning of the entire health care team. Often the nurse is expected to help coordinate the work of others, and this cannot be done without effective communication skills.

Understand the importance of accurate and complete documentation. Employers generally recognize that the new graduate must be given time to learn the documentation system used in the facility; however, the new graduate is expected to recognize the need for recording data. It is anticipated that the nurse will keep accurate, grammatically correct, and legible records that provide the necessary legal documentation of care.

Understand and have a commitment to a work ethic. This means that the employee will take the responsibility of the job seriously and will be on time, take only the allowed breaks, and will not take "sick days" unless truly ill. It also means that the new graduate recognizes that nurses may be needed 24 hours a day, 365 days a year, and that this may require sacrifices of personal convenience, such as working evening shifts or on holidays.

Possess proficiency in the basic technical nursing skills. This is an area in which a wide variety of expectations may be present. In most settings, proficiency in the basic skills is required to support activities of daily living. These skills include transferring, giving baths, and performing general hygienic measures. In some settings, nurses will be carrying out these tasks, whereas in others they will be directing or teaching others to do them, such as nursing assistants or family members. In either case, proficiency is essential to evaluate the care provided.

The technical skills or tasks that are reserved for the licensed nurse represent the area of widest diversity in the identification of essential skills. The settings in which nurses practice are diverse and, therefore, technical skills may be needed in one setting but not in another. Some facilities provide extensive orientation programs in which every skill is checked before the new graduate is allowed to proceed independently. Other employers expect the new graduate to perform the skill if able, and be checked off as required, or to ask for help if unable to be independent. Often employers are flexible in their expectations, so that it may be acceptable if an individual seems to have competency in a reasonable percentage of the skills required by that agency; further development of skill competency will be supported by the institution. Other employers have a list of skills in which competency is mandatory at the time of hire, although speed may not be expected. Also, there may be a difference between what the employer would wish and what the employer will accept.

Function with acceptable speed. This is another area where expectations differ greatly. Most employers state that they expect the new graduate will be slower; however, they may vary in how much slowness is acceptable and how soon they feel that nursing actions should become more efficient. Generally, an orientation period is planned, although the pressures on health care agencies often has shortened this considerably. An acceptable speed of function is reflected by the ability to carry out a usual licensed nurse assignment within a shift. Thus, if the usual patient care assignment for the licensed nurse is the care of five to six moderately ill patients, the new graduates are expected to accomplish this by the end of the orientation period.

IDENTIFYING POTENTIAL EMPLOYERS

It is hard to determine what expectations a new employer may have if a list of possible employers is not developed. A good starting point is to review those institutions that are familiar and gradually move outward in an ever-widening circle. An excellent example is for a student to begin with clinical sites where they worked. Often, these agencies are a known quantity. The type of care provided is familiar, as are many of their policies and procedures. Nurses who worked in a hospital as a student may even be given preference in hiring.

Another source of potential jobs is the classified section of the local newspaper. On any given day there are many job postings from small facilities as well as general recruitment announcements from larger institutions. Advertising is expensive; and, therefore, some health care agencies do not advertise and rely on those who independently seek them out as potential employers.

With electronic access, the computer resources are additional sources of potential jobs available. Many government jobs are posted on-line. Some on-line service providers have additional support services for a job search that might include career guidance or sample documents such as résumés and application letters. Usually these types of services are offered for a fee; however, they can be of great benefit during the job search.

THE APPLICATION PROCESS

If several potential employers are identified, then the new nurse needs to make an application to each of them. It is appropriate to make several job applications at the same time.

Managing the Job Search

With the changes in health care, new graduates are sometimes faced with a longer job search than anticipated. Some of the concerns that arise when this happens include: "What am I doing wrong?" "Should I work in health care in another role?" "What happens if my skills get out of date?"

Evaluating job search strategies and the letters and résumé being sent to employers is critical. It may be wise to seek assistance from a career counselor, a personal source, or professional associates. It is important to make a professional presentation.

In an effort to keep this critical job-seeking time organized and meaningful, consider the following suggestions. First, once the target organizations are identified, call the agency or hospital and obtain the name of the personnel director and double check the address to be used to mail the application. Sometimes the personnel director is not the person to whom the application letter and résumé should be mailed; there are nursing department heads who wish to review all nursing job applications submitted. It is disappointing to prepare an application and then have it lost because it was sent to the wrong address or person in the organization. The nurse should prepare applications, letters, and résumés, armed with knowledge. Gather information about prospective employers. What kind of facility is it? What types of patients do they serve, and what special services do they offer? It makes a poor impression to write a prospective employer about working in the postoperative step-down unit when that hospital does not have any step-down units.

As information about jobs begins to pile up, develop a personal record-keeping system. Some nursing recruiters suggest a file folder for each agency to which letters, applications, and résumés have been mailed. It is best to keep a typed list of each institution with the phone number, address, and name and title of the contact person. To this list add the date you sent your letter of application and résumé and notes on any information that the organization sends you.

After a résumé and letter of application are sent, make a follow-up phone call to be sure that they were received. A note to this effect should be added to the master list. When recording interviews, include the interviewer's name and the content of the interview, and dates and times of any follow-up letters or calls. Have a place to record your own notes or impressions. This will enable you to keep track of details when you manage an extensive job search. By keeping this type of record, common errors will be avoided. An inquiry letter and résumé, for example, will not be sent twice to the same agency. It is also appropriate to make a phone call or send a short note to those people who have been helpful in the past; for example, a colleague or mentor, family member, or friend who provided a job lead. This simply adds another link to the networking chain.

The Letter of Application

In today's competitive job market, it is critical that every résumé be accompanied with a letter of application, sometimes called a **cover letter**. People may present themselves positively through a well-written letter. This letter is a significant reflection of professionalism and must be prepared thoughtfully. In addition, a letter may be dealt with at the recipient's convenience, whereas a telephone call may interrupt a busy schedule. There are fewer chances for misunderstanding if your request is in writing and if you receive a written reply.

Another part of advance planning is identifying how to craft a letter focusing on any special qualifications. These should relate to the position. Additionally, each letter should be individualized to the company targetted. A form letter should not be used. Finally, the letter should be no more than one page in length but planned to present all essential information.

A good letter includes an introduction and the purpose for writing in the first paragraph so that the reader has an immediate understanding. It may also be wise to briefly state the reasons for applying for a position with this particular employer. The more specific the reason, the better the impression left. Relevant qualifications for the position should be highlighted in the next paragraph. This should not be a simple recitation of the résumé, but should either present the information in a slightly different light or add pertinent detail that is not in the résumé. If an advertisement is being responded to, each of the qualifications listed in the advertisement should be addressed. Personal skills and abilities should be related to the needs of this particular agency. If a new nurse's health care experience is limited, then he or she should state the skills gained from other jobs that would also be useful in nursing.

In the final paragraph, make a summary statement indicating why this employer should call for an interview. Ask for one. Be sure to indicate the times that will be convenient and the relevant contact information. It is also wise to indicate that a call may be forthcoming. This allows the applicant to maintain some initiative in the process. Finally, thank the person for considering the application, and close. The word "Enclosure" should appear on the bottom left. Figure 8–1 is an example of an effective cover letter.

Bear in mind that a cover letter's appearance and contents are a personal representation. People may be judged harshly on the basis of spelling, grammar, clarity, and neatness as well as on the letter's content. A letter of application should be written in standard business form, three to four paragraphs in length, on plain white or off-white business paper. Make it brief and clear. Have a first draft reviewed by a colleague or friend.

1234 Pleasant Street
Chicago, IL 60000
September 12, 2000

Thomas DiNapoli
Human Resources Manager
St. Anne's Medical Center
P.O. Box 3476
Pittsburgh, PA 15230

Dear Mr. DiNapoli:

I am applying for the position of full-time medication nurse that you advertised in the September 11 *Pittsburgh Press and Post Gazette.* My résumé is enclosed.

During the last year I worked with my health care team to establish new procedures and protocols for medication rounds. The procedures have been successfully implemented and I can bring these innovative ideas to your facility.

I would be happy to come in for an interview. I can be reached at (123) 456-7890 and will call you on September 19 to answer any questions you may have.

Sincerely,

Anita Jones, LPN

Enclosure

FIGURE 8–1 Sample cover letter

Preparing the Résumé

A **résumé** is a formal overview of a person's qualifications for a particular position. Preparing a résumé is important in a job search. Its purpose is to provide the employer with a way to quickly identify whether you have the basic qualifications for a position, and to make a personal presentation in the most positive light. The form chosen for a résumé may also be as crucial as any qualifications.

Before a form is selected, however, gather the basic data needed. These facts will need to be modified in any résumé form selected.

The résumé should provide a clear synopsis of educational and professional accomplishments. It shows a prospective employer what has been studied and where, the states in which one is licensed, and where he or she has worked. It should detail extra credentials and any other information that will land a job. Compiling the data can be a time-consuming task, though. No one wants to do it more than once. Fortunately, by using a computer, one can enter the information, then rearrange it in many different forms and for many different potential employers (Table 8–3).

Regardless of format, all résumés contain some similar information. This basic content is summarized below.

Identifying Data. The résumé always begins with a name, address, and telephone number (including area code). Usually this is at the top of the page, so a reader may easily contact an applicant. Please note: employers are not permitted to ask about age, marital status, and dependents. This information does not need to be included.

Objective. A personal goal or objective is often included. This may include both a short-term goal such as "employment as a licensed

---

TABLE 8–3
A Curriculum Vitae

Prepare professional and educational information as it occurs. With computer access, start your résumé just before graduation from nursing school. Once employed, list dates, institutions, addresses, managers, titles, functions, workshops and conferences attended with dates, certificates earned, professional memberships, degrees, continuing education courses with dates, special project assignments, etc. This begins your *curriculum vitae*, which is a complete listing of all activities related to your educational and professional career.

nurse on an adult postsurgical unit" and a long-term goal such as "with advancement to head nurse or supervisory position."

Education and Credentials. For a professional position, one should always cite one's degrees, diplomas, and the names and locations of the schools from which they were received. Include nondegree education as well. Nurses will also want to include information regarding licensure, including the license number, and other credentials. If a license is not possessed, it may be necessary to put information about when licensure is expected. Always start with the most recent degree. Include any specialty certification, when it was granted, and by whom. Finally, any special educational experiences possessed especially relate to a position, it is wise to individualize the résumé by briefly identifying those experiences.

Experience and Employment History. Employment history should be in reverse chronological order. If the traditional résumé format is used, for each job listed, include the address, dates employed, position, and duties. Even if a more skill-focused résumé format is selected that does not include details of all previous positions, this is good information to have on hand. The skill-focused résumé relates skills, responsibilities, and types of positions rather than a chronological list of employers. Be sure to include language proficiency. Computer literacy may also be a valuable skill.

Additional Experience. Volunteer and community work and awards and honors should be listed in two separate sections. Choose the items you list under volunteer and community work carefully. Your participation in community organizations, particularly service in leadership roles might be significant to an employer. This is an area that allows people to individualize their résumé to target particular skills believed to be important to the position applied for. List awards, honors, and professional associations that demonstrate competence or leadership.

References. Listing references is generally not done any longer. Most people simply place a line on the résumé that says "References available on request." Many make no mention of them at all. Most interviewers assume that a job applicant will provide references if asked.

References are typed on a separate page and given to the prospective employer if they are requested or copied onto an application form. It is important to be selective in choosing the people listed as references. Be sure to secure their permission. A primary reference is a direct employer who may easily describe work habits and effectiveness as an employee. Another good reference is an instructor or supervisor from an educational program. Some agencies request two faculty references. These people affirm an applicant's ability in the nursing field.

Once all the information is compiled, a résumé style may be selected. There are four types: chronological, functional, modified functional, and a letter. The chronological and modified functional are seen most often. The functional type does not provide enough information about work history, and a letter in lieu of an outline style is used only when you have little or no work experience related to the job you are interested in.

The choice between chronological and modified functional depends largely on how much experience one has in the field.

A chronological résumé presents information successively from current positions backwards. It is the easiest to write and the easiest to read, and probably the best choice for a new graduate. It also works well for a nurse who has a clear job target that is directly related to the work history. Figure 8–2 is an example of a chronological résumé.

A new graduate with little on-the-job experience should list educational background first. If work experience is present, begin with work history.

A modified functional résumé stresses skills, not job history. This kind of résumé works well when changing fields, for example, from staff nursing to home health care, because it permits a focus on the skills that are key to performance in the new field. Figure 8–3 is an example of a modified functional résumé.

Whichever form is adopted, be sure the vocabulary is strong. Use action verbs to describe responsibilities and experiences (Table 8–4). Language should be clear and accurate. Be sure to check spelling and grammar carefully.

Crisp, sharp, and professional are key words in describing how a résumé should appear. It should be printed on standard $8\frac{1}{2} \times 11$, white, bond paper, using a word processor with a letter quality, preferably laser, printer. Few résumés are done on a typewriter any longer; the results are just not professional.

There should be a 1-inch margin on all sides, material should be single-spaced, with double spacing between the major sections. A new graduate's résumé should not be more than one page. There is a difference of opinion among nursing recruiters about the length of résumés. Some will review a two-page résumé from an experienced nurse or a nurse executive; others believe that the one-page résumé is essential for all job applicants. Revise the résumé for each new job search. Never update it simply by adding handwritten notes.

Anita Jones, LPN
1234 Pleasant Street
Chicago, Illinois 60000
Telephone: (123) 456-7890

OBJECTIVE: Position as an LPN in long-term care setting

LICENSE NUMBER: State of Illinois #_____

**PROFESSIONAL
EXPERIENCE:**

1992–present   **General Hospital and Medical Center**
Chicago, Illinois

Position: LPN, medication nurse
Provide direct care as a team member on a 36-bed
unit.Distribute and maintain medications. Work in
cooperation with nonlicensed team members. Manage
nursing outcomes using assistive personnel. Received
three letters of commendation for patient care delivery.

1987–1992   **City Teaching Medical Center**
Chicago, Illinois

Position: LPN, general medical unit
Provided direct patient care on a 25-bed medical unit.
Gained experience caring for geriatric patients. Helped
develop unit procedures for shift rotation. Participated in
an average of 12 hours of continuing education contact
hours per year.

EDUCATION: **Chicago State University, Chicago, Illinois**
Completed 24 credit hours of course work in BSN
prerequisites, focus on physiology and psychology

Highland Community College, Freeport, Illinois
Licensed Practical Nurse, 1987
Class representative to faculty council

RELATED   Lectured 25 preschool students on keeping healthy,
EXPERIENCE: repeated program four times

AFFILIATIONS: Member, NFLPN

REFERENCES: Available upon request

FIGURE 8–2 Sample chronological résumé

Anita Jones, LPN
1234 Pleasant Street
Chicago, Illinois 60000
Telephone: (123) 456-7890

OBJECTIVE: Position as an LPN in long-term care setting

PROFESSIONAL SKILLS

Patient Care: Successfully distribute and maintain medication care for a 36-bed unit.

Patient Education: Provide all discharge teaching to patients and family caregivers. Monitor patient's skills in self-care techniques.

Administration: Set priorities and supervised nonlicensed personnel.

LICENSURE/CERTIFICATION

State of Illinois: #_____

EMPLOYMENT HISTORY

06/92–present: Medication nurse, General Hospital and Medical Center, Chicago, IL

06/90–05/92: Staff nurse, City Teaching Medical Center, Chicago, IL

EDUCATION

Chicago State University, Chicago, IL: completed 24 credit hours in BSN prerequisites.

LPN, Highland Community College, Freeport, IL

PROFESSIONAL ORGANIZATIONS

Member, NFLPN

REFERENCES

Available upon request.

FIGURE 8–3 Sample modified functional résumé

TABLE 8–4			
Action Verbs for Résumé Use			
accelerated	designed	influenced	performed
accomplished	developed	initiated	pinpointed
achieved	directed	instructed	planned
adapted	effected	interpreted	proficient in
administered	eliminated	launched	programmed
analyzed	established	lectured	proposed
approved	evaluated	led	proved
completed	expanded	maintained	provided
conceived	expedited	managed	recommended
conducted	facilitated	mastered	reduced
controlled	found	motivated	reinforced
coordinated	generated	operated	reorganized
created	implemented	organized	revamped
delegated	improved	originated	reviewed
demonstrated	increased	participated	revised
Additional action verbs:			
scheduled	solved	supervised	trained
set up	streamlined	supported	translated
simplified	structured	taught	utilized

The Electronic Résumé

A growing number of employers are now using "automated applicant tracking systems," databases that electronically store, compare, and retrieve résumés of prospective employees. In fact, health care recruiters in hospitals, managed care organizations, long-term care facilities, cancer rehabilitation centers, and home health agencies are finding new nurses through résumé databases and career centers on the Internet (Figure 8–4).

An automated applicant tracking system works much like automated systems used for literature searches. Résumés are compiled in a database, and the employer uses keywords, or specific criteria to search the database for information needed. The tracking system then retrieves those résumés entered into the database that contain the keywords specified.

Anita Jones, LPN
1234 Pleasant Street
Chicago, Illinois 60000
Telephone: (123) 456-7890

Keyword Summary: Nursing. Health Care. Medication Administration. LPN. Med/Surg. Spanish. NFLPN. Relocation.

OBJECTIVE: Position as an LPN in a long-term care setting.

LICENSE NUMBER: State of Illinois: #_____

EXPERIENCE:

1992–present: *MEDICATION NURSE*, 450+–bed medical center, Chicago, IL

Distribute and maintain medications. Coordinate care with team members on a 36-bed unit. Supervise nonlicensed personnel.

1987–1992   *STAFF NURSE*, 450+–bed medical center, Chicago, IL

Provide direct patient care. Help patients perform activities of daily living. Experience with geriatric patients.

EDUCATION: Chicago State University, Chicago, IL
Coursework toward a BSN.

LPN, Highland Community College, Freeport, IL, 1987

AFFILIATIONS: NFLPN

PERSONAL: Fluent in Spanish. Willing to relocate.

REFERENCES: Available on request

FIGURE 8–4 Sample electronic résumé

Depending on how sophisticated the system is, the screen may display a list of résumé "titles" or header lines for each résumé. The employer can then select the résumés of choice and view them as full text or in an applicant summary—a short, standard fact sheet that the system creates by extracting certain relevant data from the whole résumé.

Some employers have their own, in-house automated applicant tracking system. Any résumés they receive by mail are electronically scanned and stored in the company's database. When a position opens up, the recruiter logs on to the tracking system to search for a candidate.

The Interview

A job interview is one of the adventures in one's professional life. The interview should be a two-way conversation in which you will be gaining as well as giving information. Current job interviews vary in format depending on the management style of the person responsible for the interview process or the policies of the organization. Because of this diversity, be prepared for whatever the interview may bring.

Before going to the interview, many nurses outline information that they want to obtain and questions that they want answered. A good strategy involves writing questions so that they are clearly stated and they are not forgotten in the tense atmosphere that often exists in an interview situation. Time spent reflecting on personal views in advance will be valuable during the interview.

When planning for an employment interview, it is important to consider one's appearance, attitude, and approach, as well as the content of the interview. Personal appearance will likely evoke some type of response from the interviewer. Consider what that response should be and dress appropriately. Being neat and well-groomed contributes to a businesslike atmosphere. Make a conscious decision about the impression desired. Although some may wish that appearances had no effect on the opinions of others, remember that, in reality, appearance often does make a significant difference.

Take to the interview a file that contains the following material: professional license, cardiopulmonary resuscitation card, hepatitis B vaccinations, and TB skin test results that are less than 12 months old. Take a copy of the résumé to the interview for reference. In addition, be prepared with the names, addresses, and telephone numbers of all references, as well as one's own Social Security number. Take along a black pen to complete any forms, and a notepad with questions. Have a place to make personal notes of important information obtained during the interview. This increases self-confidence if questions about statements on the résumé arise during an interview.

Many organizations have leveled interviews. The initial interview may only be the first of several. Some organizations have the personnel director do the initial interview. If that goes well, then the applicant may be called back to interview with the nurse manager, and a third interview may take place with members of the nursing staff. This type of process is rigorous and often tests the applicant's desire for the job. The prospective employer wants to see if the applicant has the stamina and commitment to continue through the process. Another reason for leveled interviews is to give numerous people, who could be future coworkers, an opportunity to meet and learn more about the applicant. It gives everyone the opportunity to interact with one another and assists in determining if this job is a good fit. This process should be seen as a great opportunity.

The single- or double-interview process is much more manageable. This occurs when one interviews with only one or several people. The committee interview is also common and one applicants should be psychologically prepared to do. Look at the group, being sure to make eye contact with each individual. Make sure that the role of each person present is understood. Write down individual names and roles on a notepad and then review the list. This allows an applicant to direct a question to a specific individual or to use an individual's name when responding to a question. While replying to the person who asks the question, glance at others as you make your point.

Manner in the interview is also important. Although the employer expects the applicant to be nervous, he or she will be interested in whether nervousness makes the applicant unable to respond appropriately. Follow common rules of courtesy. Wait to be asked to sit down before you take a chair. Avoid any distracting mannerisms, such as chewing gum or fussing with your hair, face, or clothes. Be serious when appropriate, but do not forget to smile and be pleasant. The interviewer is also thinking of the impact an applicant will make on patients, visitors, and other staff members.

Role-playing an interview with a friend or relative may build confidence. Another technique is to visualize the interview situation and mentally rehearse responses to questions. Many interviewers focus on asking questions about past experiences and future plans. Others focus their questions on specific accomplishments and problems encountered in past nursing experiences. Presenting hypothetical problems for consideration, and asking for appropriate nursing responses are common. Applicants should be adept at responding to scenarios and case studies. The best resources are management books written for licensed nurses.

There are some legal aspects of a job interview that are important to know and understand. It is illegal for an interviewer to ask any questions about age, ethnic background, birthplace, religion, credit rating, sexual preference, number of dependents and their ages, pregnancy, or child care arrangements. If the interviewer asks a question that is illegal, such as a question regarding age or marital status, it might be wise to redirect the question to address what appears to be the concern of the interviewer. For example, in response to a question about age a good reply might be: "Perhaps you believe that I appear to be young and inexperienced. I want to assure you that I have demonstrated my maturity and responsibility both in my nursing education and in my position with my previous employer." Avoid simple yes or no answers, and try to describe or explain in order to give a more complete picture.

An interview usually covers a wide variety of subjects. The interviewer may direct the flow of topics or may encourage the applicant to bring up his or her issues. Applicants who focus initial attention on the issues of wages and benefits may be viewed as more concerned about themselves than about nursing. If asked to present questions, ask professional questions first. Make sure they are appropriate for the interviewer. In the personnel department, ask about the overall mission and philosophy of the organization, its organizational structure, and how authority and accountability are determined. With a nursing interviewer, however, demonstrate concern about how nursing care is given and by whom, where authority and responsibility for nursing care decisions lie, the philosophy underlying care, and the availability of continuing education. Before leaving, be sure to cover such topics as hours, schedules, pay scales, and benefits.

Applicants sometimes feel at a loss as to exactly what is being asked. Before proceeding they should seek clarification, but must be careful that their manner of asking does not offend the interviewer. A clarifying approach is to state clearly what is perceived to be the central question before continuing. "To be clear, you would like me to identify a situation in which I believe I responded effectively to a problem. Is that correct?"

If unfamiliar with the interview process, read a few books on the topic. Reading several different books will provide a variety of viewpoints. It may provide strategies that are more comfortable.

Interview Follow-up Procedures

Any initial inquiry should be followed-up. If an interview was involved, follow-up with a letter. If an interview was not involved, continue to contact the potential employer at intervals in order to learn of other job opportunities. An applicant's "eagerness" usually strikes employers favorably, although it is important not to be ""too eager."

After the interview, write a brief thank-you letter. Figure 8–5 provides an example of a thank-you letter. If it was a group interview, direct the letter to the person who seemed to be in charge. In that letter, thank the individual for the time and attention. Restate any agreement you feel was reached. For example, "I understand that I am to call your office next week to learn whether I have been scheduled for an interview with the maternity unit manager." Close the letter with a positive comment about the organization. Even if not offered a job, this approach leaves a positive impression.

1234 Pleasant Street
Chicago, IL 60000
September 12, 2000

Thomas DiNapoli
Human Resources Manager
St. Anne's Medical Center
P.O. Box 3476
Pittsburgh, PA 15230

Dear Mr. DiNapoli:

Thank you for taking the time to speak with me yesterday about the position of medication nurse at St. Anne's Medical Center. I was very impressed with your company, and the job sounds wonderful. I'm more than ever convinced that my experience can benefit your company.

I appreciated the opportunity to meet you and learn about St. Anne's.

Sincerely,

Anita Jones, LPN

FIGURE 8–5 Sample thank-you note

PROFESSIONAL LIABILITY INSURANCE

Many nurses disagree about the need for professional liability insurance. They assume the coverage provided by their employer is adequate; however, as the discussion in Chapter 4 related, this may be a misconception.

Nurses claim to be competent and knowledgeable in their area of practice. The health care consuming public, therefore, holds nurses accountable for their practice. As a result, all too frequently nurses are named as defendants in malpractice lawsuits against hospitals, physicians, and health care agencies. Employers are to some extent responsible for the actions of their employees; however, this responsibility stops when the employee leaves works. Additionally, if the nurse violates policy and the employer is required to pay damages, the employer has the right to sue the nurse to recover the damages.

Some experts believe that having malpractice insurance simply invites lawsuits. These experts also believe that the best protection against litigation is quality nursing practice. Nevertheless, it can be argued that malpractice insurance is a must for all nurses, regardless of the area of clinical practice. Additionally, some nurses find it comforting to have their own attorney because the agency's attorney will be representing the agency and protecting the agency's interest, not the nurse's.

There are two basic types of liability protection: the occurrence policy and the claims made policy. Occurrence policies protect the nurse against events that take place during the period of time the policy is active, even if a claim is filed after the policy is terminated. The claims made policy protects the nurse against claims made during the time the policy is in effect. If a claim is made after the policy is terminated, the nurse is not covered. Clearly, occurrence policies seem to offer better protection for the nurse.

How much coverage should a nurse buy? That is difficult question at best. Some insurance carriers no longer offer a $500,000 policy because of the larger settlements currently being awarded, and they report that nurses are requesting $1,000,000 to $1,500,000 policies. The costs for liability insurance policies can range from $70 to $200, depending on the type of coverage purchased and the area of clinical practice. It is advised to shop wisely and to remember that costs can be higher with advanced clinical practice or for nurses who work in critical care areas in acute care hospitals. For example, nurse practitioners, nurse midwives, nurse anesthetists, intensive care and coronary care nurses, and neonatal intensive care nurses may need policies with larger amounts of coverage, and the cost for the greater coverage is usually higher.

Liability insurances for nurses are somewhat similar in the basics but may differ in other areas. For example, a liability policy may include personal liability coverage, which means the nurse could be covered for non-nursing incidents.

There are some important questions to ask before purchasing liability coverage and a list of them is provided in Table 8–5. When purchasing insurance coverage, it is essential to read the policy and make sure all issues are clearly understood. Finally, the nurse should validate the company's reputation. Before the decision to purchase is completed, request information from several companies so that policies can be reviewed and compared. It is well worth the time to find the company that provides the coverage that offers the best protection.

If employment status is changed, the insurer should be notified in writing. Retain a copy of the notification letter. Some nursing experts recommend sending important notifications via registered mail so that a receipt of delivery is provided to the sender. The insurer should also be informed of any incidents that may lead to litigation. When in doubt, insurers may be contacted for advice about an incident or an

TABLE 8–5

Questions to Ask Before Purchasing Liability Insurance

- What are the financial limitations of the policy?
- Who is covered?
- Under what conditions is the policy renewable?
- What is the annual premium cost?
- How long does the coverage last?
- Does the policy provide occurrence or claims made coverage?
- When am I covered? On the job or off the job?
- Am I provided with an attorney?
- Is my salary guaranteed while I am in court?
- Are all the defense costs covered?
- Am I required to settle?
- What other items are included in the coverage?

CAREER TIP

Choice of Attorney

Some insurers do not permit the nurse's choice of an attorney; the company will decide who the attorney is. Additionally the insurer can decide that an attorney is not needed, or the insurer may decide to settle the case. Many nurses believe that settling a case is an automatic indication of guilt. These are questions that must be answered before insurance coverage is purchased.

issue that needs clarification. When calling the insurer, have the policy number available and make a record of the conversation—what was said, who said it, and the date and time of the conversation. Any written correspondence should always include full name and policy number.

Should a nurse decide to cancel his or her policy, closely follow the procedures outlined in the policy for cancellation. Return the policy, including a letter indicating the date the coverage should end. Nurses must compare the costs and benefits of having professional liability insurance against the cost of potential legal fees and loss of personal assets.

N-CLEX EXAMINATION

To assist boards of nursing in making licensure decisions for practical/vocational nurse and registered nurse candidates, the National Council of State Boards of Nursing created the N-CLEX-PN examination and the N-CLEX-RN examination. These two legally defensible and psychometrically sound examinations measure the competencies needed to perform safely and effectively as an entry-level practical/vocational or registered nurse. The National Council Examination Committee oversees the development of these examinations. This entails several crucial steps, beginning with reviewing the results of the job analysis studies to the creation of quality test questions.

The National Council conducts licensed practical/vocational nurse (LPN/VN) and registered nurse (RN) job analysis studies every three years. These studies are designed to collect data from newly licensed nurses that describe what they actually do on the job. All recommended revisions to the test plans are presented to National Council's membership, which includes all state and territorial boards of nursing, for approval.

The N-CLEX-PN and the N-CLEX-RN identify the essential content and distribution of test questions that are included on the respective examinations. The test plan serves as the link between entry-level practice and the examination itself.

The current N-CLEX-PN Test Plan, developed from the 1997 Job Analysis of Newly Licensed, Practical/Vocational Nurses, includes the patient needs categories and percentage of test questions as displayed in Table 8–6.

Legally defensible and psychometrically sound N-CLEX examination items (test questions) require extensive development and evaluation

TABLE 8–6

N-CLEX-PN Test Plan

Categories	Percentage of Test Questions
A. Safe, Effective Care Environment	
1. Coordinated Care	6–12%
2. Safety and Infection Control	7–13%
B. Health Promotion and Maintenance	
3. Growth and Development through the Life Span	4–10%
4. Prevention and Early Detection of Disease	4–10%
C. Psychosocial Integrity	
5. Coping and Adaptation	6–12%
6. Psychosocial Adaptation	4–10%
D. Physiological Integrity	
7. Basic Care and Comfort	10–16%
8. Pharmacological Therapies	5–11%
9. Reduction of Risk Potential	11–17%
10. Physiological Adaptation	13–19%

methods. The examination committee participates throughout the item development process from approving the appointment item writers (the nursing experts who write the test questions), to developing the test plan and giving final approval of examination items prior to their inclusion in the master pool. This intricate process ensures the integrity of N-CLEX examination items that accurately measure the competencies needed to perform effectively and safely as an entry-level practical/vocational or registered nurse.

The state boards use the results of the examination to determine whether a license will be issued to an applicant. New graduates proceed through the steps for application to take the examination through their individual nursing education programs. The nursing school will complete certain required forms indicating that applicants have successfully completed the nursing education program.

The N-CLEX tests knowledge of patient need such as physiologic and psychological needs, safety, and health promotion, as well as nursing process, including data collection, planning, and implementation. The test is administered via a computer using a method called computerized adaptive testing (CAT); the computer selects the test questions as a person takes the examination. All of the questions must be answered in the order they are presented and questions cannot be skipped. The examination is in a multiple choice format and candidates must correctly answer a minimum of 85 questions and a maximum of 205 questions during the maximum 5-hour testing period.

There are only two keys on the computer keyboard to be concerned with, the ENTER key and the SPACE BAR key. All other keys are turned off and do not affect the examination. The SPACE BAR key is used to move through the answer options. The ENTER key allows the candidate to record the answer. When an answer is recorded, the computer automatically progresses to the next question. At the testing site, each candidate is given an orientation to the computer and will go through a keyboard practice/orientation process. Every effort is made to make sure that the candidate understands and is comfortable with the testing procedures.

Computer Adaptive Testing

In August 1991, the Assembly of the National Council voted to implement computer adaptive testing (CAT) for the national licensure examinations. This was decided after extensive research and field testing to determine the validity and reliability of computer testing. A licensure examination must be able to measure the competencies required for safe practice and distinguish consistently between candidates who demonstrate those competencies and those who do not.

In April 1994, the National Council of State Boards of Nursing, Inc. implemented CAT for the N-CLEX for both practical/vocational nurses (N-CLEX-PN) and registered nurses (N-CLEX-RN). This represented a major advance in the implementation and administration of the examination.

With CAT, each candidate receives a different set of questions via the computer. The computer develops an exam that is unique to the individual candidate. The questions to be presented to the candidate are determined by the response of the candidate to the previous question. The number of questions each candidate receives and the testing time for each candidate will vary. The exam is adapted to the individual candidate who is taking it. The questions presented will continue to reflect the N-CLEX plan based on the nursing process, patient needs, and the job analysis studies (Table 8–7).

"Field test" questions will be integrated into the exam. These are questions that allow the NCSBN examination committee to gather statistical information to determine whether a question is valid and can be added to the test bank of questions for future selection. These

TABLE 8–7

The Technical Aspects of the N-CLEX

- All questions are multiple choice with four options. Some questions stand alone and others relate to a situation or background information.
- All of the information needed for each question is available on the screen.
- If needed, scratch paper will be provided and it must be turned in.
- There is only one answer to each question, and there is no partial credit.
- Calculators are not permitted.
- All questions must be answered; another question will not appear until the one on the screen is answered.
- You not be able to go back to a previous question once that question has been removed from the screen.
- If you need to take a break, notify one of the testing staff.

ASK YOURSELF

The nurse practice act, or state board rules and regulations require that LP/VNs work under the direction of an RN, physician, or dentist. In some states, the language in the regulations indicates "other health care providers" can supervise the LP/VN. Specifically, who are the other health care providers? In the state in which you are practicing, are you required to follow orders written by nurse practitioners? Physician assistants? The answers can vary by individual states and it is essential to know who can direct your practice.

questions are not counted in the grading of the examination, and time has been allocated for the candidate to answer them.

The results are mailed to the candidate by the state board within two to four weeks after the examination. Applicants may retake the examination; however, the National Council requires a waiting period of ninety-one days between testings. Individual state boards may have additional regulations regarding retaking the examination. With successful passage of the N-CLEX-PN, a license is issued from the state board. It is the licensed nurse's responsibility to maintain the license according to individual state requirements. Additionally, the licensed nurse must notify the state board, in writing, of any changes in name and address.

Preparing for the NCLEX

Nursing schools will typically advise students as to the specific dates the forms are due at the state office. The directions should be followed exactly. The state boards do not respond favorably to applications that are not submitted on time or are submitted in an incorrect format. If a new nurse wishes to apply for licensure in another state, it is usually his or her responsibility to contact the board of nursing in that state to obtain the necessary forms.

Review courses that may assist in organizing study materials and identifying areas where additional help is needed are a very valuable course of action. The percentage of graduates passing the examination is higher for those who participate in either a formal review class or who initiate a structured study plan.

It is usually not required to take a formal review class; however, some nursing schools offer a two- to three-day review course to the graduating class as a part of the basic educational preparation. If it is offered, take advantage of it. Also, many nursing schools will provide an assessment test shortly before graduation. These tests are graded and the results are returned to the school before graduation. The results may include not only the test scores in specific areas of study, but may indicate specific areas of focus where additional study is needed. Many of these testing services will also provide a list of textbooks with specific page references for study. Some nursing schools provide these tests as an additional reference to assist graduates in developing a structured study plan.

Although an outside formal review class is not required, a structured plan of study is essential. Set a study schedule that is realistic. Two to three hours a day for two or three days a week is realistic; eight hours a day on a single day off is not an effective plan. Personal style should influence the number of hours per study session, the frequency of the scheduled sessions, and the amount of research that is required. Some people study best alone, whereas others prefer groups. If a study group is preferred, make sure that the group agrees on a particular plan that will fit everyone's needs.

When planning a study schedule, utilize a calendar to record days of the week, hours, and subject areas. Place priority on those areas that require the most help. Many nursing educators advise and encourage their students to purchase review books not only for study but for the test banks that are available. Many of the review books have computer disks, which is advantageous, because it allows the graduate to be exposed to the computer before taking the N-CLEX examination. N-CLEX review materials are also moving onto the Internet. Additionally, the review books have rationales for the correct answer and for the incorrect answers. This is an excellent learning and a very strong review tool for graduates.

Many nursing instructors think that approximately 1,500 to 2,000 test questions be answered during the study preparation. This allows the graduate to become familiar with the language and the phrasing of the test items (questions). Also, it permits the development and refinement of test-taking strategies. Using the strategies outlined in Table 8–8, nurses may proceed through the testing with an organized approach and often perform better as a result.

TABLE 8–8

Test-Taking Strategies

- Read the stem (question) carefully.
- Do not overanalyze the question.
- Focus on *what* is being asked.
- Identify the patient. The patient can be a visitor or a family member.
- Evaluate all the options in a systematic manner.
- Eliminate options you know are incorrect.
- Do not look for the *correct* answer among the options (answers). Look for the answer that is *most* appropriate.
- Keep in mind the nursing process and Maslow's hierarchy of needs.
- Presume that you have ideal supplies and equipment in patient care situations.
- Read, do not scan, the question carefully, looking for *key* words such as *essential, required, first, must, necessary, primary, early,* and *best.*

Many nursing educators advise students to wait until after graduation before they start to study for the N-CLEX examination. The requirements for graduation will probably be very time consuming and there may not be sufficient time or energy to commit to a study schedule. Also, the time may be needed to study for final examinations for school and information "overload" may be an issue.

Some recent graduates who successfully completed the examination recommend a minimum of four to six weeks of study preparation. This recommendation should take into consideration the factors discussed before (the number of hours per session, the frequency, the amount of subject areas to cover, and personal style). Some graduates study for longer periods and others use a shorter period of time. Some graduates work immediately after graduation and work schedules must also be considered.

When test bank questions are utilized as an integral component of the N-CLEX preparation, the percentage of correct answers may be an indicator of examination readiness. Nursing educators suggest a passing percentage of 80% consistently as an indicator for appropriate preparation. Whatever indicator selected, the prime time to take the examination is when the test taker is confident and prepared.

KEY POINTS

- Mentoring and networking are important strategies to assist in the transition from student to graduate.
- Each nurse must be familiar with the nurse practice act for the state in which he or she is practicing.
- It is essential to be aware of basic entry-level competencies because these are the expectations of potential employers.
- In the job search, maintaining an organized, written plan is important.
- The cover letter, or letter of application, is necessary to accompany the résumé.
- The résumé should be tailored to meet the current position of interest.
- A curriculum vitae should be maintained on a computer, if there is access; this allows for easy maintenance.
- The curriculum vitae should be used to create various résumés for different positions.
- A structured study plan is important in preparing to take the N-CLEX examination.
- Nurses differ in their opinions regarding liability insurance however, each nurse should make an individual decision.
- It is the responsibility of the licensed nurse to maintain the nursing license according to the regulations of the state in which he or she practices.

CRITICAL THINKING ACTIVITIES

1. Write your short- and long-term goals with a plan on how you can achieve these goals.
2. Develop personal strategies for managing reality shock. Include the rationale for each strategy.
3. Make an appointment with a nursing manager, a personnel director, or a nursing executive for a job interview. Ask for an evaluation of the interview to assist you in developing your interviewing skills.
4. Based on your perception of the needs in your community, write a mission statement for a hospital that would serve the needs of the area.

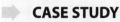
CASE STUDY

You are three months from graduating from an accredited LP/VN program and you are excited about your upcoming role as a licensed nurse. You have decided that you want to work in a hospital for one or two years in an effort to polish your clinical skills and have role models and mentors available to you. You have had clinical experience in a local 300-bed hospital that is appealing for you to consider it as a place of employment.

Describe how you may determine in which area of the hospital you want to work, and how you are going to make an application to the hospital.

Case Study Suggestions

The area in which you choose to apply for a position depends on your career goals. It is a reasonable consideration to want to work in an area where you may have many opportunities to improve your clinical skills, but you need to ask yourself which skills. Do you want to be great at care of adults, children, or families? Your career plan determines your optimum place to work. After you have identified which area is for you, be alert to available positions on that unit. Do you know anyone who works there and who could serve as a part of your network? If you do, take that person to lunch or to the cafeteria for a quiet moment to discuss the possibilities for you and your wish to be employed there.

BIBLIOGRAPHY

Bozell, J. (1999). *Anatomy of a job search—a nurse's guide to finding and landing the job you want.* Philadelphia: Springhouse.

Deluca, M. J., & Deluca, N. F. (1997). *Wow! Resumes for creative careers.* New York: McGraw-Hill.

Farber, G. (1995). Job hunting in the world of nursing. *Nursing World.* *42*(1), 21–22.

Green, L. A. (1991b). Life insurance: Vital protection for your vital signs, Part II: Health care trends and transition. *Nursing, 99,* 116–121.

Krannich, C. R., & Krannich, R. L. (1997). *201 dynamite job search letters* (3rd ed.). New York: Impact Publishers.

INTERNET RESOURCES

http://www.career-skills.com/Home.htm
http://www.uwec.edu/Admin/Career/lab/interview.html
http://www.qwuincareers.com/tntvres.html
http://www.drjohnholleman.com/fall/carintdr.html

Appendices

APPENDIX A: NAPNES STANDARDS OF PRACTICE FOR LICENSED PRACTICAL/VOCATIONAL NURSES

The LP/VN provides individual and family-centered care. The LP/VN shall:

A. Utilize principles of nursing process in meeting specific patient needs of patients of all ages in the areas of:
  1. Safety
  2. Hygiene
  3. Nutrition
  4. Medication
  5. Elimination
  6. Psycho-social and cultural
  7. Respiratory needs

B. Utilize appropriate knowledge, skills and abilities in providing safe, competent care.

C. Utilize principles of crisis intervention in maintaining safety and making appropriate referrals when necessary.

D. Utilize effective communication skills.
  1. Communicate effectively with patients, family members of the health team, and significant others.
  2. Maintain appropriate written documentation.

E. Provide appropriate health teaching to patients and significant others in the areas of:
  1. Maintenance of wellness
  2. Rehabilitation
  3. Utilization of community resources

F. Serve as a patient advocate:
  1. Protect patient rights
  2. Consult with appropriate others

The LP/VN fulfills the professional responsibilities of the practical/vocational nurse. The LP/VN shall:

A. Know and apply the ethical principles underlying the profession.

B. Know and follow the appropriate professional and legal requirements.

C. Follow the policies and procedures of the employing institution.

D. Cooperate and collaborate with all members of the health care team to meet the needs of family-centered nursing care.

E. Demonstrate accountability to his/her nursing actions.

F. Maintain currency in terms of knowledge and skills in the area of employment.

The LP/VN follows the NAPNES code of ethics. The LP/VN shall:

1. Consider as a basic obligation the conservation of life and the prevention of disease.

2. Promote and protect the physical, mental, emotional, and spiritual health of the patient and his family.

3. Fulfill all duties faithfully and efficiently.

4. Function within established legal guidelines.

5. Accept personal responsibility (for his/her acts) and seek to merit the respect and confidence of all members of the health team.

6. Hold in confidence all matters coming to his/her knowledge, in the practice of his profession, and in no way at no time violate this confidence.

7. Give conscientious service and charge just remuneration.

8. Learn and respect the religious and cultural beliefs of his/her patient and of all people.

9. Meet his/her obligation to the patient by keeping abreast of current trends in health care through reading and continuing education.

10. As a citizen of the United States of America, uphold the laws of the land and seek to promote legislation which shall meet the health needs of its people.

(Reprinted with permission of National Association for Practical/Vocational Nurses)

APPENDIX B: NFLPN NURSING PRACTICE STANDARDS FOR THE LICENSED PRACTICAL/VOCATIONAL NURSE

Preface

The Standards were developed and adopted by the NFLPN to provide a basic model whereby the quality of health service and nursing service and nursing care given by LP/VNs may be measured and evaluated.

These nursing practice standards are applicable in any practice setting. The degree to which individual standards are applied will vary according to the individual needs of the patient, the type of health care agency or services and the community resources.

The scope of licensed practical nursing has extended into specialized nursing services. Therefore, specialized fields of nursing are included in this document.

The Code for Licensed Practical/Vocational Nurses

The Code, adopted by NFLPN in 1961 and revised in 1979, provides a motivation for establishing, maintaining and elevating professional standards. Each LP/VN, upon entering the profession, inherits the responsibility to adhere to the standards of ethical practice and conduct as set forth in this section.

1. Know the scope of maximum utilization of LP/VN as specified by the nursing practice act and function within this scope.
2. Safeguard the confidential information acquired from any source about the patient.
3. Provide health care to all patients regardless of race, creed, cultural background, disease, or lifestyle.
4. Refuse to give endorsement to the sale and promotion of commercial products or services.
5. Uphold the highest standards in personal appearance, language, dress, and demeanor.
6. Stay informed about issues affecting the practice of nursing and delivery of health care and, where appropriate, participate in government and policy decisions.
7. Accept the responsibility for safe nursing by keeping oneself mentally and physically fit and educationally prepared to practice.
8. Accept responsibility for membership in NFLPN and participate in its efforts to maintain the established standards of nursing practice and employment policies which lead to quality patient care.

INTRODUCTORY STATEMENT

Definition

Practical/Vocational nursing means the performance for compensation of authorized acts of nursing which utilize specialized knowledge and skills and which meet the health needs of people in a variety of settings under the direction of qualified health professionals.

Scope

Practical/Vocational nursing comprises the common core of nursing and, therefore, is a valid entry into the nursing profession.

Opportunities exist for practicing in a milieu where different professions unite their particular skills in a team effort for one common objective—to preserve or improve an individual patient's functioning.

Opportunities also exist for upward mobility within the profession through academic education and for lateral expansion of knowledge and expertise through both academic and continuing education.

STANDARDS

Education

The Licensed Practical/Vocational Nurse:

1. Shall complete a formal education program in practical nursing approved by the appropriate nursing authority in the state.
2. Shall successfully pass the National Council Licensure Examination for Practical Nurses.
3. Shall participate in initial orientation within the employing institution.

Legal/Ethical Status

The Licensed Practical/Vocational Nurse:

1. Shall hold a current license to practice nursing as an LP/VN in accordance with the law of the state wherein employed.
2. Shall know the scope of nursing practice authorized by the Nursing Practice Act in the state wherein employed.
3. Shall have a personal commitment to fulfill the legal responsibilities inherent in good nursing practice.
4. Shall take responsible actions in situations wherein there is unprofessional conduct by a peer or other health care provider.

5. Shall recognize and have a commitment to meet the ethical and moral obligations of the practice of nursing.
6. Shall not accept or perform professional responsibilities which the individual knows (s)he is not competent to perform.

Practice

The Licensed Practical/Vocational Nurse:

1. Shall accept assigned responsibilities as an accountable member of the health care team.
2. Shall function within the limits of educational preparation and experience as related to the assigned duties.
3. Shall function with other members of the health care team in promoting and maintaining health, preventing disease and disability, caring for and rehabilitating individuals who are experiencing an altered health state, and contributing to the ultimate quality of life until death.
4. Shall know and utilize the nursing process in planning, implementing, and evaluating health services and nursing care for the individual patient or group.
   a. Planning: The planning nursing includes:
      1) Assessment of health status of the individual patient, the family and community groups.
      2) An analysis of the information gained from assessment.
      3) The identification of health goals.
   b. Implementation: The plan for nursing care is put into practice to achieve the stated goals and includes:
      1) Observing, recording and reporting significant changes which require intervention or different goals.
      2) Applying nursing knowledge and skills to promote and maintain health, to prevent disease and disability and to optimize functional capabilities of an individual patient.
      3) Assisting the patient and family with activities of daily living and encouraging self-care as appropriate.
      4) Carrying out therapeutic regimens and protocols prescribed by an RN, a physician, or other person authorized by state law.
   c. Evaluations: The plan for nursing care and its implementations are evaluated to measure the progress toward the stated goals and will include appropriate persons and/or groups to determine:

1) the relevancy of current goals in relation to the progress of the individual patient
2) the involvement of the recipients of care in the evaluation process
3) the quality of the nursing action in the implementation of the plan.
4) a re-ordering of priorities or new goal setting in the care plan.

5. Shall participate in peer review and other evaluation processes.
6. Shall participate in the development of policies concerning the health and nursing needs of society and in the roles and functions of the LP/VN.

Continuing Education

The Licensed Practical/Vocational Nurse:

1. Shall be responsible for maintaining the highest possible level of professional competence at all times.
2. Shall periodically reassess career goals and select continuing education activities which will help to achieve these goals.
3. Shall take advantage of continuing education opportunities which will lead to personal growth and professional development.
4. Shall seek and participate in continuing education activities which are approved for credit by appropriate organizations, such as the NFLPN.

Specialized Nursing Practice

The Licensed Practical/Vocational Nurse:

1. Shall have had at least 1 year's experience in nursing at the staff level.
2. Shall present personal qualifications that are indicative of potential abilities for practice in the chosen specialized nursing area.
3. Shall present evidence of completion of a program or course that is approved by an appropriate agency to provide the knowledge and skill necessary for effective nursing services in the specialized field.
4. Shall meet all the standards of practice as set forth in this document.

(Reprinted with permission of the National Federation of Licensed Practical Nurses—www.nflpn.org)

APPENDIX C: NURSING-RELATED ORGANIZATIONS

	Year Established	Membership Eligibility	Publications (monthly unless otherwise noted)
Overall Professional Organizations			
American Nurses Association (ANA) 600 Maryland Avenue, SW Suite 100 West Washington, DC 20024-2571	1896	RNs only	*American Journal of Nursing; The American Nurse* (for others, write for list)
International Council of Nurses (ICN) 3, Place Jean Marteau 1201 Geneva 20, Switzerland	1900	National professional nurse organization	*International Nursing Review*
National Federation of Licensed Practical Nurses, Inc. 893 Hwy. 70 W Garner, NC 27529		All LPNs or LVNs	
National Federation of Specialty Nursing Organizations (NFSNO) 875 Kings Highway West Deptford, NJ 08096		Specialty nursing organizations	
National League for Nursing (NLN) 350 Hudson Street New York, NY 10014	1952	Individuals and agencies interested in the profession of nursing and delivery of nursing care	*Nursing and Health Care Perspectives* (for others, write for list)

	Year Established	Membership Eligibility	Publications (monthly unless otherwise noted)
Overall Professional Organizations *continued*			
National Student Nurse Association (NSNA) 555 West 57th Street, Suite 1327 New York, NY 10019	1953	Officially enrolled students of RN and RN baccalaureate programs	*Imprint* (5 times/year)
Organizations Related to Scholarship and Leadership in Nursing			
Alpha Tau Delta 5207 Mesada Street Alta Loma, CA 91737	1921	Students in baccalaureate programs in nursing	*Captions of Alpha Tau Delta* (biennial)
American Academy of Nursing (AAN) c/o American Nurses Association 600 Maryland Ave., SW Suite 100 West Washington, DC 20024-2571	1973	Members elected by current members, based on contribution to nursing; use title "Fellow" (FAAN)	*Nursing Outlook* (bimonthly)
Sigma Theta Tau International 550 West North Street Indianapolis, IN 46202-3163	1922	High achievers; senior students in baccalaureate, master's, and doctoral programs; outstanding RNs with baccalaureate or higher degree	*Image, Reflections* (newsletters, quarterly)

	Year Established	Membership Eligibility	Publications (monthly unless otherwise noted)
Groups Related to Ethnic/Racial Origin			
American Indian Nurses Association (AINA) P.O. Box 1588 Norman, OK 73071	1972	Student nurses and RNs of American Indian ancestry	*Newsletter of the AINA* (bimonthly)
Association of Black Nursing Faculty (ABNF) Inc. 1708 North Roxboro Road Durham, NC 27701		Nursing faculty members of African-American background and those interested in their issues	
National Association of Hispanic Nurses 1501 Sixteenth St., NW Washington, DC 20036	1976	Hispanic nurses, associate/all nurses	Newsletter (quarterly)
National Black Nurses Association, Inc. 1012 Tenth Street, NW Washington, DC 20001-4492	1971	African-American RNs	*Journal of National Black Nurses' Association* (twice yearly)
Philippine Nurses Association of America, Inc. P.O. Box 10200 San Diego, CA 92120		Filipino nurses and those inter-ested in their issues	

	Year Established	Membership Eligibility	Publications (monthly unless otherwise noted)
Educationally Oriented Associations			
American Association of Colleges of Nursing (AACN)	1969	Collegiate program with upper-division major in nursing	*Journal of Professional Nursing* (bimonthly); *AACN Newsletter* (10 times/yr); (write for list)
Council on Collegiate Education for Nursing for the Southern Regional Education Board (SREB) 1340 Spring Street, NW Atlanta, GA 30309	1963	Colleges and universities in the southern states that have nursing programs	(write for list)
Mid-Atlantic Regional Nursing Association (MARNA) 350 Hudson Street New York, NY 10014	1981	Agencies preparing persons in health care and that deliver health care	*Marnagram* (quarterly)
Midwest Alliance in Nursing, Inc. (MAIN) 2251 East 46th Street, Suite E-3 Indianapolis, IN 46205	1979	Agencies engaged in providing direct nursing care or teaching person to provide direct nursing care	*MAINlines* (bimonthly newsletter)

	Year Established	Membership Eligibility	Publications (monthly unless otherwise noted)
National Association for Practical Nurse Education and Service, Inc.	1941	All persons interested in LPN/LVN education	*Journal of Practical Nursing* (quarterly); *NAPNES Forum*
National Council of State Boards of Nursing (NCSBN) 676 N St. Clair Suite 550 Chicago, IL 60611-2921	1978	State/territorial licensing boards	*Issues*
National Organization for Associate Degree Nursing (NOADN) 1730 North Lynn Street Suite 502 Arlington, VA 22209-2004	1985	Open	*Advancing Clinical Care*
North American Nursing Diagnosis Association (NANDA) 1211 Locust Street Philadelphia, PA 19107	1976	RNs	*Nursing Diagnoses*
Western Institute of Nursing (WIN) P.O. Drawer P Boulder, CO 80302	1957	Colleges and universities that have nursing programs	(write for list)

Occupational or Specialty-Related Organizations

Academy of Medical Surgical Nurses East Holly Ave., Box 56 Pitman, NJ 08071			
American Academy of Ambulatory Care Nursing East Holly Ave., Box 56 Pitman, NJ 08071	1974	RNs in administration of ambulatory nursing	

	Year Established	Membership Eligibility	Publications (monthly unless otherwise noted)
Occupational or Specialty-Related Organizations *continued*			
American Academy of Nurse Practitioners Capitol Station, LBJ Bldg. P.O. Box 12846 Austin, TX 78711		Registered nurses in advanced practice as nurse practitioners	
American Association for the History of Nursing, Inc. P.O. Box 90803 Washington, DC 20003	1980	Anyone interested in the history of nursing	*The Bulletin* (4 times/yr)
American Association of Critical Care Nurses (AACN) 101 Columbia Aliso Viejo, CA 92656-1491	1969	RNs, LPNs, student nurses	*Critical Care Nursing Focus on Critical Care* (bimonthly)
American Association of Diabetes Educators 600 North Michigan Avenue Suite 1400 Chicago, IL 60661		Individuals engaged in educating those with diabetes	
American Association of Legal Nurse Consultants 4700 West Lake Avenue Glenview, IL 60025			
American Association of Nurse Anesthetists (AANA) 200 South Prospect Avenue Park Ridge, IL 60068-4001	1931	RNs who are certified registered nurse anesthetists (CRNAs)	*American Association of Nurse Anesthetists Journal* (bimonthly); *AANA Bulletin* (bimonthly)

	Year Established	Membership Eligibility	Publications (monthly unless otherwise noted)
The American Association of Nurse Attorneys (TAANA) 720 Light Street Baltimore, MD 21230-3826	1982	Nurses who are attorneys or are in law school and attorneys in nursing schools	*Inside TAANA* (newsletter, quarterly)
American Association of Occupational Health Nurses (AAOHN), Inc. 50 Lenox Pointe Atlanta, GA 30324-3176	1942	RNs practicing in an occupational health setting	*AAOHN Journal; AAOH News*
American Association of Office Nurse Consultants 109 Kinderkamack Rd. Montvale, NJ 07645			
American Association of Spinal-Cord Injury Nurses 75-20 Astoria Blvd. Jackson Heights, NY 11370-1178	1983	RNs and LPNs who practice in diverse SPCI settings	*SCI Nursing* (quarterly journal); also educational and practice guidelines
American Burn Association Burn Treatment Center Crozier-Chester Medical Center 15th and Upland Avenue Chester, PA 19013		Professionals working with burn patients	
American College of Nurse Midwives (ACNM) 818 Connecticut Avenue NW Suite 900 Washington, DC 20006	1955	RNs who are certified nurse midwives or students in accredited programs	*Journal of Nurse Midwifery Quickening* (newsletter)

	Year Established	Membership Eligibility	Publications (monthly unless otherwise noted)
Occupational or Specialty-Related Organizations *continued*			
American Holistic Nurses Association 401 Lake Boone Trail, Suite 201 Raleigh, NC 27607	1981	Active: RN, LPN/LVN Contributing: all others	*Journal of Holistic Nursing* (annual); *Beginnings* (newsletter); *Journal of Neuroscience Nursing* (bimonthly)
American Nephrology Nurses Association (AANA) North Woodbury Road, Box 56 East Holly Avenue Pitman, NJ 08071	1969	RNs, LVNs employed in the field	*Journal of ANNA* (6 times/yr); *AANA Update* (newsletter)
American Organization of Nurse Executives (AONE) 325 Seventh St., NW Suite 700 Washington, DC 20036		RNs in administrative positions	
American Psychiatric Nurses' Association 1200 Nineteenth St., NW Suite 300 Washington, DC 20036			
American Public Health Association (APHA) Public Health Nursing Section 1015 15th Street, NW Washington, DC 20005	1972	All persons interested in public health Various categories of membership available	*American Journal of Public Health; The Nation's Health*

	Year Established	Membership Eligibility	Publications (monthly unless otherwise noted)
American Radiological Nurses Association 2021 Spring Road Suite 600 Oakbrook, IL 60521	1981	Active: RNs employed in radiologic nursing Associate: other RNs and LPNs in radiologic nursing	*ARNA Images* (4 times/yr)
American Society for Long-Term Care Nurses 660 Lonely Cottage Drive Upper Black Eddy, PA 18972-9313	1990	Anyone interested in supporting long-term care	*ASLTCN Journal* (bimonthly)
American Society of Ophthalmic Registered Nurses (ASORN), Inc. P.O. Box 193030 San Francisco, CA 94119	1976	RNs working in ophthal-mology	*Insight* (newsletter)
American Society of Pain Management Nurses 1550 So. Coast Highway Suite 201 Laguna Beach, CA 92651		Student and corporate membership available	*ASPMN Pathways* (quarterly newsletter)
American Society for Parenteral and Enteral Nutrition—Nurses' Committee 8630 Fenton Street, Suite 412 Silver Springs, MD 20910-3803	1975	Multidiscipli-nary profes-sionals working with parenteral and enteral nutrition	

	Year Established	Membership Eligibility	Publications (monthly unless otherwise noted)
Occupational or Specialty-Related Organizations *continued*			
American Society of Plastic and Reconstructive Surgical Nurses, Inc. East Holly Rd., Box 56 Pitman, NJ 08071	1975	Active: RNs, LPNs working in the field Associate: RNs, LPNs interested in the field	*Journal of Plastic and Reconstructive Surgical Nursing*
American Society of Post-Anesthesia Nurses 6900 Groove Road Thorofare, NJ 08086	1980	RNs, LPNs, anesthesiologists, CRNAs	*Breathline Journal of Post Anesthesia Nursing* (quarterly)
American Urological Association Allied 11512 Allecingie Parkway, Ste C Richmond, VA 23235	1972	Active: RNs, LPNs, PAs, technicians Associate: industry, physicians	*AUAA Journal* (quarterly); *Urogram* (newsletter)
Association for Practitioners in Infection Control 505 East Hawley Street Mundelein, IL 60060			
Association of Nurses in AIDS Care (ANAC) 704 Stoney Hill Road, Suite 106 Yardley, PA 19067 (215) 321-2371 http://www.mc.vanderbilt.edu/adl/pathfinders/missions/anac.html	1988	Nurses, industry, and affiliates interested in promoting health, welfare, and rights of HIV-infected persons	*Journal of Association of Nurses in AIDS Care (JANAC)*; *ANACdotes* (quarterly newsletter)

	Year Established	Membership Eligibility	Publications (monthly unless otherwise noted)
Association for Professionals in Infection Control and Epidemiology 1016 16th Street NW Washington, DC 20036	1972	Active: professionals in infection control Associate: other	*APIC* (bimonthly) (for others, write for list)
Association for the Care of Children's Health 3615 Wisconsin Avenue, NW Washington, DC 20016	1965	All individuals interested in children's health	*Children's Health Care* (for others, write for list)
Association of Operating Room Nurses (AORN) 2170 South Parker Road Suite 300 Denver, CO 80231-5711	1949	Active: RNs employed in OR or related education program or in research	*AORN Journal*
Association of Pediatric Oncology Nurses 4700 West Lake Road Glenview, IL 60025-1485	1976	RNs	*APON News-letter* (quarter-ly) (for others, write for list)
Association of Rehabilitation Nurses 4700 West Lake Road Glenview, IL 60025-1485	1974	Regular: RNs Associate: all interested persons	*Rehabilitation Nursing* (bimonthly journal); pamphlets
Association of Women's Health, Obstetric, and Neonatal Nurses (AWHONN) (Formerly NAACOG) 700 14th Street NW, Suite 600 Washington, DC 20005 (202) 662-1600	1969	RNs and allied health individuals in OGN nursing	*Journal of Obstetric, Gynecologic and Neonatal Nursing* (JOGN) (bimonthly); *AWHONN Newsletter*

	Year Established	Membership Eligibility	Publications (monthly unless otherwise noted)
Occupational or Specialty-Related Organizations *continued*			
Coalition of Nurse Practitioners, Inc. P.O. Box 123 East Greenbush, NY 12061	1980	Nurse practitioners and students in nurse practitioner programs	*Coalition Communique* (quarterly)
Department of School Nurses of the National Education Association (NEA) 1201 Sixteenth Street, NW Washington, DC 20036	1968	School nurse members of the NEA	*The School Nurse*
Dermatology Nurses' Association East Holly Avenue, Box 56 Pitman, NJ 08071-0056	1981	Active: RNs, LPNs/LVNs involved in dermatology	*DNA Focus* (bimonthly newsletter)
Developmental Disabilities Nurses' Association 1720 Willow Creek Circle, Suite 515 Eugene, OR 97402			
Drug and Alcohol Nursing Association 660 Lonely Cottage Drive Upper Black Eddy, PA 18972	1979	Active: nurses caring for clients with drug- and alcohol-related disorders Associate: all others	*DANA Newsletter* (quarterly)
Emergency Nurses Association (ENA) 216 Higgins Road Park Ridge, IL 60068	1970	RNs	*The Journal of Emergency Nursing; Emergency Nursing Care Curriculum*

	Year Established	Membership Eligibility	Publications (monthly unless otherwise noted)
Flight Nurse Section Aerospace Medical Association Washington National Airport Washington, DC 20001	1964	Designated flight nurses and RNs who are members of Aerospace Medical Association	*Aviation, Space, and Environmental Medicine*
Hospice Nurses Association 5512 No. Umberland Street Pittsburgh, PA 15217-1131			
International Association for Enterostomal Therapy (IAET), Inc. 2081 Business Center Drive Suite 290 Irvine, CA 92715	1968	Active: graduates of accredited IAET program	*Journal of Enterostomal Therapy*
Intravenous Nurses' Society, Inc. 2 Brighton Street Belmont, MA 02178	1973	Nurses interested in intravenous therapy	*Journal of Intravenous Therapy*
National Alliance of Nurse Practitioners 325 Pennsylvania Ave., SE Washington, DC 20003-1100		DONS in long-term care agencies	
National Association of Directors of Nursing Administration in Long Term Care (NADONA/LTC) 10999 Reed Hartman Hwy., Suite 229 Cincinnati, OH 45242			
National Association of Health Care Recruitment P.O. Box 5769 Akron, OH 44372	1975	Active: health care recruiters	*Recruitment Directions* (10 times/yr)

	Year Established	Membership Eligibility	Publications (monthly unless otherwise noted)
Occupational or Specialty-Related Organizations *continued*			
National Association of Neonatal Nurses 1304 Southpoint Blvd. Suite 280 Petaluma, CA 94954	1984	Regular: RNs Associate: all others	*Neonatal Network: The Journal of Neonatal Nursing* (bimonthly)
National Association of Orthopaedic Nurses East Holly Avenue, Box 56 Pitman, NJ 08071	1980	RNs, LPNs, LVNs	*Orthopaedic Nursing* (for others, write for list)
National Association of Nurse Practitioners in Reproductive Health 325 Pennsylvania Avenue, SE Washington, DC 20003			
National Association of Pediatric Nurse Associates/Practitioners (NAPNAP) 1101 Kings Highway North, Suite 206 Cherry Hill, NJ 08034	1973	RNs with advanced education who are primary care practitioners in pediatrics	*The Pediatric Nurse Practitioner* (newsletter); *The Journal of Pediatric Health Care*
National Association of Physicians' Nurses 900 South Washington St. Suite G-13 Falls Church, VA 22046			

	Year Established	Membership Eligibility	Publications (monthly unless otherwise noted)
National Association of School Nurses Lamplighter Lane, P.O. Box 1300 Scarborough, ME 04074	1969	Active: RNs employed by educational institutions Other categories for students, retirees, organizations	*School Nurse Journal NAS*; *Newsletter* (quarterly)
National Flight Nurses Association 6900 Groove Road Thorofare, NJ 08086-9447	1981		*Aeromedical Journal* (bimonthly); *Across the Board* (quarterly)
National Gerontological Nurses Association 7250 Parkway Drive, Suite 510 Hanover, MD 21076		Other categories for students, retirees, organizations	
National Nurses Society on Addiction 4101 Lake Boone Trail Suite 201 Raleigh, NC 27607	1983	Regular: RNs Associate: all others	*Annual Review of Nursing in the Addictions* (quarterly newsletter)
Nurse Consultants Association, Inc. 414 Plaza Drive, Suite 209 Westmont, IL 60559	1979	RNs with 60% of income from consultant-type sources	Quarterly newsletter; annual membership directory

	Year Established	Membership Eligibility	Publications (monthly unless otherwise noted)
Occupational or Specialty-Related Organizations *continued*			
Nurses Organization of Veterans' Affairs 1726 M Street NW Suite 1101 Washington, DC 20034			
Oncology Nursing Society 501 Holiday Drive Pittsburgh, PA 15220		Nurses interested in oncology	
Respiratory Nursing Society 4700 West Lake Avenue Glenview, IL 60025-1485			
Society for Vascular Nursing (SVN) 309 Winter Street Norwood, MA 02062	1982	Active: currently licensed nurses	*SVN Journal* (quarterly)
Society of Gastroenterology Nurses and Associates, Inc. 401 North Michigan Avenue Chicago, IL 60611	1974	Individuals employed as gastrointestinal nurses or assistants	*Gastroenterology Nursing* (bimonthly)
Society of Otorhinolaryngology and Head-Neck Nurses, Inc. 116 Canal Street, Suite A New Smyrna Beach, FL 32168	1976	RNs actively working in ORL/head-neck nursing	*ORL-Head and Neck Nursing* (4 times/yr); *Update* (quarterly newsletter)
Society of Pediatric Nurses 7250 Parkway Drive Suite 510 Hanover, MD 21076			

	Year Established	Membership Eligibility	Publications (monthly unless otherwise noted)
Transcultural Nursing Society College of Nursing Madonna University 36600 Schoolcraft Rd. Livonia, MI 48150	1979	Nurses and non-nurses	Biannual newsletter
World Federation of Neuroscience Nurses P.O. Box 3703 Parramotta, NSW 2150 Australia		Professional nurses working in neuroscience	

Miscellaneous

	Year Established	Membership Eligibility	Publications (monthly unless otherwise noted)
American Assembly for Men in Nursing 437 Twin Bay Drive Pensacola, FL 32534-1350	1971	All those supportive of concerns of men in nursing	*Interaction*
National Nurses for Life 1998 Menold Allison Park, PA 15104			
Nurses Christian Fellowship 6400 Schroeder Road P.O. Box 7895 Madison, WI 53707	1948	Christian students and RNs	*Journal of Christian Nursing* (quarterly)
Nurses Educational Funds 555 West 57th Street New York, NY 10019	1911	Donors welcome	Semiannual newsletter
Nurses' House, Inc. 350 Hudson Street New York, NY 10014	1925	Payment of annual contribution	

APPENDIX D: NURSING LICENSING AUTHORITIES (BOARDS OF NURSING) UNITED STATES AND U.S. TERRITORIES

Note: For specific information regarding licensure requirement, regulations, and fees, contact the specific licensing authority. Current addresses, telephone numbers, and directors can also be obtained on the Internet through the National Council of State Boards of Nursing at:

http://www.ncsbn.org/pfiles/mbdirect.html

Alabama
Alabama Board of Nursing
P.O. Box 303900
Montgomery AL 36130
Phone: (334) 242-4060
Fax: (334) 242-4360
Judi Crume, Executive Officer

Alaska
Alaska Board of Nursing
Dept. of Comm. & Econ. Development
Div. of Occupational Licensing
3601 C Street, Suite 722
Anchorage, AK 99503
Phone: (907) 269-8161
Fax: (907) 562-5781
Dorothy Fulton, Executive Director

American Samoa
American Samoa Health Services
Regulatory Board
LBJ Tropical Medical Center
Pago Pago, AS 96799
Phone: (684) 633-1222
Fax: (684) 633-1027
Marie Ma'o, Director, Nursing Services

Arizona
Arizona State Board of Nursing
1651 East Morten Avenue, Suite 150
Phoenix, AZ 85020
Phone: (602) 255-5902
Fax: (602) 255-5130
Joey Ridenour, Executive Director

Arkansas
Arkansas State Board of Nursing
University Tower Building
1123 South University, Suite 800
Little Rock, AR 72204
Phone: (501) 686-3350
Fax: (501) 686-2714
Faith Fields, Executive Director

California
California Board of Registered Nursing
P.O. Box 944210
Sacramento, CA 94244
Phone: (916) 322-3350
Fax: (916) 327-4402
Ruth Ann Terry, Executive Director

California Board of Vocational Nurse
   and Psychiatric Technician Examiners
2535 Capitol Oaks Drive, Suite 205
Sacramento, CA 95833
Phone: (916) 263-7800
Fax: (916) 263-7859
Teresa Bello-Jones, Executive Director

Colorado
Colorado Board of Nursing
1560 Broadway, Suite 670
Denver, CO 80202
Phone: (303) 894-2430
Fax: (303) 894-2821
Karen Brumley, Program Administrator

Connecticut
Connecticut Department of Public
   Health Board of Examiners for
   Nursing
410 Capitol Avenue, MS 12NUR
P.O. Box 340308
Hartford, CT 06134
Phone: (860) 509-7624
Fax: (860) 509-7650
Marie Hilliard, Executive Officer

Delaware
Delaware Board of Nursing
Cannon Building, Suite 203
P.O. Box 1401
Dover, DE 19903
Phone: (302) 739-4522
Fax: (302) 739-2711
Iva Boardman, Executive Director

District of Columbia
District of Columbia Board of Nursing
614 H. Street NW
Washington, DC 20001
Phone: (202) 727-7468
Fax: (202) 727-7662
Barbara Hagans, Contact Person

Florida
Florida Board of Nursing
4080 Woodcock Drive, Suite 202
Jacksonville, FL 32207
Phone: (904) 858-6940
Fax: (904) 858-6964
Marilyn Bloss, Executive Director

Georgia
Georgia Board of Nursing
166 Pryor Street, SW
Atlanta, GA 30303
Phone: (404) 656-3943
Fax: (404) 657-7489
Shirley Camp, Executive Director

Georgia State Board of Licensed
    Practical Nurses
166 Pryor Street, SW
Atlanta, GA 30303
Phone: (404) 656-3921
Fax: (404) 651-9532
Patricia Swann, Executive Director

Guam
Guam Board of Nurse Examiners
P.O. Box 2816
Agana, GU 96910
Phone: (671) 475-0251
Fax: (671) 477-4733
Teofila Cruz, Nurse Examiner
    Administrator

Hawaii
Hawaii Board of Nursing
P.O. Box 3469
Honolulu, HI 96801
Phone: (808) 586-2695
Fax: (808) 586-2689
Kathleen Yokouchi, Executive Officer

Idaho
Idaho Board of Nursing
P.O. Box 83720
Boise, ID 83720
Phone: (208) 334-3110
Fax: (208) 334-3262
Sandra Evans, Executive Director

Illinois
Illinois Department of Professional
    Regulation
James R. Thompson Center
100 West Randolph, Suite 9-300
Chicago, IL 60601
Phone: (312) 814-2715
Fax: (312) 814-3145
Jacqueline Waggoner, Nursing Act
    Coordinator

Illinois Department of Professional
    Regulation
320 West Washington St., 3rd Floor
Springfield, IL 62786
Phone: (217) 785-9465
Fax: (217) 782-7645
Mary Jo Southard, Chief Testing Officer

Indiana
Indiana State Board of Nursing
Health Professions Bureau
402 W. Washington St., Suite 401
Indianapolis, IN 46204
Phone: (317) 232-2960
Fax: (317) 233-4236
Laura Langford, Executive Director

Iowa
Iowa Board of Nursing
State Capitol Complex
Des Moines, IA 50319
Phone: (515) 281-3255
Fax: (515) 281-4825
Lorinda Inman, Executive Director

Kansas
Kansas State Board of Nursing
Landon State Office Building
900 SW Jackson, Suite 551
Topeka, KS 66612
Phone: (913) 296-4929
Fax: (913) 296-3929
Patsy Johnson, Executive Administrator

Kentucky
Kentucky Board of Nursing
312 Wittinton Parkway, Suite 300
Louisville, KY 40222
Phone: (502) 329-7000
Fax: (502) 329-7011
Sharon Weisenbeck, Executive Director

Louisiana

Louisiana State Board of Nursing
3510 North Causeway Blvd., Suite 501
Metairie, LA 70002
Phone: (504) 838-5332
Fax: (504) 838-5349
Barbara Morvant, Executive Director

Louisiana State Board of Practical
  Nurse Examiners
3421 N. Causeway Blvd., Suite 203
Metairie, LA 70002
Phone: (504) 838-5791
Fax: (504) 838-5279
Terry DeMarcay, Executive Director

Maine

Maine State Board of Nursing
24 Stone Street
State House Station #158
Augusta, ME 04333
Phone: (207) 287-1133
Fax: (207) 287-1149
Jean Caron, Executive Director

Maryland

Maryland Board of Nursing
4140 Patterson Avenue
Baltimore, MD 21215
Phone: (410) 764-5124
Fax: (410) 358-3530
Donna Dorsey, Executive Director

Massachusetts

Massachusetts Board of Registration
  in Nursing
Leverett Saltonstall Building
100 Cambridge Street, Room 1519
Boston, MA 02202
Phone: (617) 727-9961
Fax: (617) 727-2197
Theresa Bonanno, Executive Director

Michigan

Bureau of Occupational and
  Professional Regulation
Michigan Department of Consumer
  and Industry Services
Ottawa Towers N., 611 West Ottawa
Lansing, MI 48933
Phone: (517) 373-9102
Fax: (517) 373-2179
Carol Johnson, Licensing Administrator
  (Board Support Section)

Office of Testing Services
Michigan Department of Commerce
P.O. Box 30018
Lansing, MI 48909
Phone: (517) 373-3877
Fax: (517) 335-6696
Kara Schmitt, Director, OTS

Minnesota

Minnesota Board of Nursing
2700 University Avenue, Wes #108
St. Paul, MN 55114
Phone: (612) 642-0567
Fax: (612) 642-0574
Joyce Schowalter, Executive Director

Mississippi

Mississippi Board of Nursing
239 North Lamar Street, Suite 401
Jackson, MS 39201
Phone: (601) 359-6170
Fax: (601) 359-6185
Marcia Rachel, Executive Director

Missouri

Missouri State Board of Nursing
P.O. Box 656
Jefferson City, MO 65102
Phone: (573) 751-0681
Fax: (573) 751-0075
Florence Stillman, Executive Director

Montana

Montana State Board of Nursing
111 North Jackson
P.O. Box 20051
Helena, MT 59620
Phone: (406) 444-2071
Fax: (406) 444-7759
Dianna Wickham, Executive Director

Nebraska

Professional and Occupational
  Licensure Division
Nebraska Department of Health
P.O. Box 94986
Lincoln, NE 68509
Phone: (402) 471-4376
Fax: (402) 471-3577
Charlene Kelly, Section Administrator

Nevada
Nevada State Board of Nursing
P.O. Box 46886
Las Vegas, NV 89114
Phone: (702) 739-1575
Fax: (702) 739-0298
Lonna Burress, Executive Director

New Hampshire
New Hampshire Board of Nursing
Health and Welfare Building
Concord, NH 03301
Phone: (603) 271-2323
Fax: (603) 271-6605
Doris Nuttelman, Executive Director

New Jersey
New Jersey Board of Nursing
P.O. Box 45010
Newark, NJ 07101
Phone: (201) 504-6586
Fax: (201) 648-3481

New Mexico
New Mexico Board of Nursing
4206 Louisiana Boulevard, NE
Suite A
Albuquerque, NM 87109
Phone: (505) 841-8340
Fax: (505) 841-8347
Nancy Twigg, Executive Director

New York
New York State Board of Nursing
State Education Department
Cultural Education Center, Room 3023
Albany, NY 12230
Phone: (518) 474-3843
Fax: (518) 473-0578
Milene Sower, Executive Secretary

Northern Mariana Islands
Commonwealth Board of Nurse
    Examiners
Public Health Center
P.O. Box 1458
Saipan, MP 96950
Phone: (670) 234-8950
Fax: (670) 234-8930
Elizabeth Torres-Untalan, Chairperson

North Carolina
North Carolina Board of Nursing
P.O. Box 2129
Raleigh, NC 27602
Phone: (919) 782-3211
Fax: (919) 781-9461
Carol Osman, Executive Director

North Dakota
North Dakota Board of Nursing
919 South 7th Street, Suite 504
Bismarck, ND 58504
Phone: (701) 328-9777
Fax: (701) 328-9785
Ida Rigley, Executive Director

Ohio
Ohio Board of Nursing
77 South High Street, 7th Floor
Columbus, OH 43266
Phone: (614) 466-3947
Fax: (614) 466-0388
Dorothy Fiorino, Executive Director

Oklahoma
Oklahoma Board of Nursing
2915 North Classen Blvd., Suite 524
Oklahoma City, OK 73106
Phone: (405) 525-2076
Fax: (405) 521-6089
Sulinda Moffett, Executive Director

Oregon
Oregon State Board of Nursing
800 NE Oregon Street, Box 25
Suite 465
Portland, OR 97232
Phone: (503) 731-4745
Fax: (503) 731-4755
Joan Bouchard, Executive Director

Pennsylvania
Pennsylvania State Board of Nursing
P.O. Box 2649
Harrisburg, PA 17105
Phone: (717) 783-7142
Fax: (717) 787-0250
Mariam Limo, Executive Secretary

Puerto Rico
Commonwealth of Puerto Rico
Board of Nurse Examiners
Call Box 10200
Santurce, PR 00908
Phone: (787) 725-8161
Fax: (787) 725-7903
Luisa Colom, Executive Director

Rhode Island
Rhode Island Board of Nursing
    Registration and Nursing Education
Cannon Health Building
Three Capitol Hill, Room 104
Providence, RI 02908
Phone: (401) 277-2827
Fax: (401) 277-1272
Carol Lietar, Executive Officer

South Carolina
South Carolina State Board of Nursing
Executive Center Drive, Suite 220
Columbia, SC 29210
Phone: (803) 731-1648
Fax: (803) 731-1647
Margaret Johnson, Interim Executive
    Director

South Dakota
South Dakota Board of Nursing
3307 South Lincoln Avenue
Sioux Falls, SD 57105
Phone: (605) 367-5940
Fax: (605) 367-5945
Diana Vander Woude, Executive
    Secretary

Tennessee
Tennessee State Board of Nursing
426 Fifth Avenue North
1st Floor — Cordell Hull Building
Nashville, TN 37247
Phone: (615) 532-5166
Fax: (615) 741-7899
Elizabeth Lund, Executive Director

Texas
Texas Board of Nurse Examiners
P.O. Box 140466
Austin, TX 78714
Phone: (512) 305-7400
Fax: (512) 305-7401
Katherine Thomas, Executive Director

Texas Board of Vocational Nurse
    Examiners
William P. Hobby Bldg., Tower 3
333 Guadalupe Street, Suite 3-400
Austin, TX 78701
Phone: (512) 305-8100
Fax: (512) 305-8101
Marjorie Bronk, Executive Director

Utah
Utah State Board of Nursing
Division of Occupational and
    Professional Licensing
P.O. Box 45805
Salt Lake City, UT 84145
Phone: (801) 530-6628
Fax: (801) 530-6511
Laura Poe, Executive Administrator

Vermont
Vermont State Board of Nursing
109 State Street
Montpelier, VT 05609
Phone: (802) 828-2396
Fax: (802) 828-2484
Anita Ristau, Executive Director

Virgin Islands
Virgin Islands Board of Nursing
    Licensure
P.O. Box 4247
Verterans Drive Station
St. Thomas, VI 00803
Phone: (809) 776-7397
Fax: (809) 777-4003
Winifred Garfield, Executive Secretary

Virginia
Virginia Board of Nursing
6606 West Broad Street, 4th Floor
Richmond, VA 23230
Phone: (804) 662-9909
Fax: (804) 662-9943
Nancy Durrett, Executive Director

Washington
Washington State Nursing Quality
    Assurance Commission
Department of Health
P.O. Box 47864
Olympia, WA 98504
Phone: (360) 753-2686
Fax: (360) 586-5935
Patty Hayes, Executive Director

West Virginia

West Virginia State Board of Examiners
for Practical Nurses
101 Dee Drive
Charleston, WV 25311
Phone: (304) 558-3572
Fax: (304) 558-4367
Nancy Wilson, Executive Secretary

West Virginia Board of Examiners for
Registered Professional Nurses
101 Dee Drive
Charleston, WV 25311
Phone: (304) 558-3596
Fax: (304) 558-3666
Laura Skidmore Rhodes, Executive
Secretary

Wisconsin

Wisconsin Department of Regulation
and Licensing
1400 East Washington Avenue
P.O. Box 8935
Madison, WI 53708
Phone: (608) 266-2112
Fax: (608) 267-0644
Thomas Neumann, Administrative
Officer

Wyoming

Wyoming State Board of Nursing
2020 Carey Avenue, Suite 110
Cheyenne, WY 82002
Phone: (307) 777-7601
Fax: (307) 777-3519
Toma Nisbet, Executive Director

Glossary

accreditation a process involving a program voluntarily seeking a review by a given organization to determine whether the program meets preestablished criteria of that organization.

advance directives signed documents to be followed if a patient becomes unresponsive or incompetent. The documents specify what treatment(s) the patient would choose to accept or refuse if able to do so.

advocacy protection and support of another's rights.

ambulatory care ambulatory care centers stress convenience and they are open at times other than traditional office hours. Nurses provide technical skills, determine priority of patient care needs, and patient education. An urgent care center that provides walk-in emergency care services is a special type of ambulatory care center.

appeal a request for a review and/or retrial of legal issues.

approved program a program that meets minimum standards set by the respective state agency responsible for overseeing educational programs.

autonomy the respect we have for others as human beings, which allows them the right to make judgments and choose actions.

beneficence the duty to do good to others, to help them, and to further their interests.

breach of duty the failure to conform to the standard of practice, thus creating a risk for a person that a reasonable person would have foreseen.

case management a process of coordinating an individual patient's health care for the purpose of maximizing positive outcomes and containing costs.

civil law concerned with relationships among people and the protection of a person's rights.

community-based health care care that is provided to people who live within a defined geographic region or have common needs.

confidentiality respecting privileged information and maintaining privacy of information.

consumer a consumer is someone who uses a commodity or service.

content knowledge information learned from written documents, through interactions with others, and through nursing practice.

controlling checking that plans are being carried out as planned and evaluating the outcomes of the actions.

cover letter an application letter used as a written introduction and accompanies a résumé.

crime any wrong punishable by the state.

cultural competence congruent behaviors, attitudes, and policies that come together in a system so the professionals can work effectively in a cross-cultural situation.

cultural diversity in nursing addressing the differences among all people who require specific knowledge and skills for safe and effective care.

culturally sensitive care nursing care that is appropriate for the patient within the context of the patient's beliefs, values, and specific care needs.

culture shock the individual is stunned by cultural differences and even immobilized until he or she is able to work through the feelings related to the vastly different nature of the alien culture.

curriculum vitae a complete written record of all activities related to one's educational and professional career.

defendant the person at whom the complaint is directed.

deposition an out-of-court, under-oath statement of a witness.

diagnostic-related groups a prospective payment plan that pays the health care provider a predetermined, fixed amount that is determined by the medical diagnosis or specific procedure.

directing involves supervision and ongoing decision making to carry out the plans.

directive leadership describes a leader who makes all the decisions and tells staff what to do.

discovery pretrial procedure allowing one party to examine vital witnesses and/or documents held exclusively by the adverse party.

duty the relationship between the plaintiff (the person bringing the suit) and the defendant (the person being sued).

fidelity keeping promises.

habits accepted ways of doing things that work, save time, or are necessary.

health a condition of physical, mental, and social well-being and the absence of disease or other abnormal conditions.

health maintenance organizations prepaid group health care plans that allow enrollees to receive all the medical services they require

through a group of affiliated providers.

holistic of or pertaining to the whole; considering all factors in the approach to patient care.

illness an abnormal process in which aspects of the social, emotional, or intellectual condition and function of a person are diminished or impaired.

informed consent the patient's right to self-determination about the care he or she will receive.

inpatient people who enter a hospital and stay for more than 24 hours are said to be inpatients.

inquiry examining issues in depth and questioning that which may seem immediately obvious.

in-service education educational classes offered to nurses at their place of employment.

interrogatories written questions taken from or asked of witnesses before the scheduled trial.

justice refers to justified distribution of benefits and risks/burdens in a community and can underlie principles of access, distribution, and appropriateness of care.

leadership the ability to influence others to strive for a vision or goal, or to change.

leveled interview several interviews by various people at different positions in the organization.

liability legal concept that one is responsible and will be held accountable for one's actions (personal liability).

litigation a lawsuit.

long-term care long-term care centers are designed to provide care for periods ranging from days to years. Settings providing long-term care are ususaly independent facilities, but they may be associated with a hospital. Examples include nursing homes, retirement facilities, and residential institutions.

malpractice in law, professional negligence that is the proximate cause of injury or harm to a patient, resulting from a lack of professional knowledge, experience, or skill that can be expected in others in the profession or from a failure to exercise reasonable care or judgment in the application of professional knowledge, experience, or skill. Malpractice is failure to meet a professional standard of care.

managed care an organized system of health care that influences the selection and use of high-quality and cost-effective health care services of a population. Model of nursing care delivery in which the primary nurse uses a predetermined critical pathway to establish and monitor the extent and timing of care within an anticipated length of hospital stay.

management a systematic process of getting the job done or accomplishing a goal by planning, organizing, directing, and controlling.

Medicaid a federally funded program established under Title 19 of the Social Security Act. It is a federally funded public assistance program for people with low incomes.

Medicare a national and state health insurance program for the elderly under Title 18.

mentor a mentor is a more skilled or more experienced person who serves as a role model, teaches, sponsors, encourages, counsels, and befriends a less skilled or less experienced person for the purpose of promoting the latter's personal and/or professional development.

NANDA The North American Nursing Diagnosis Association.

negligence the commission of an act that a prudent person would not have done or the omission of a duty that a prudent person would

have fulfilled resulting in injury or harm to another person. Failure to meet the ordinary standards of care, one not involving special knowledge or skill, which leads to harm.

networking method of informing people about your goals or desires in an informal manner.

nonmaleficence avoid causing harm.

organizing arranging work to be done in small units so that it can be accomplished.

outpatient a person who requires health care services but does not need to stay in an institution for those services. Patients receive treatment, care, education and are then sent home.

paradigm originally a scientific term, commonly used to mean a model, theory, perception, assumption, or frame of reference.

participative leadership describes the leader who involves staff in problem solving, goal setting, and decision making.

patient a person, family, group, or community.

plaintiff the complaining party in a lawsuit.

planning an ongoing process to decide what to do, when, where, how, by whom, and with what resources.

preferred provider organization (PPO) an organization that allows third-party payers, such as insurance companies, to contract with a group of health care providers to provide services at a lower fee in return for prompt payment and a guaranteed volume of patients and services.

primary health care a community-based strategy that focuses on simple, local, inexpensive solutions to health problems through universal access and affordability of health care, health of the population, and consumer involvement.

primary nursing method of nursing care delivery in which a registered nurse assumes responsibility for developing a 24-hour nursing plan of care and for integrating that plan with the therapy plan of the other health care professionals.

public health agency local, state, or federal agencies that provide public health services to members of various communities.

reality shock reality shock occurs when the new graduate feels that it is impossible to administer the quality of nursing care needed within the limitations of the current health care system.

rehabilitation centers these centers specialize in services for patient requiring physical or emotional rehabilitation and for treatment of any type of drug dependency.

refresher class educational classes offered to nurses who wish to bring themselves up to date in current trends of nursing.

résumé an overview of one's qualifications for a position.

standards of care acts permitted to be performed or prohibited from being performed by a prudent person working within the parameters of his or her training, license, and experience and the conditions existing at the time; the nurse's duty to a patient with whom there is an established nurse-patient relationship to provide reasonable, prudent care required by the circumstances.

stereotyping assuming conformity to a major pattern. Expecting people to act in a characteristic manner without regard to individual characteristics.

team nursing a team of nursing personnel cares for a group of patients, with team members assigned specific care functions or procedures to perform for all the patients.

tort category of law involving civil wrongs against another's person or property; torts include negligence, false imprisonment, assault, battery, defamation, invasion of privacy, and fraud.

veracity telling the truth.

voluntary agencies community agencies are often nor-for-profit organizations that are financed by donations, grants, and fundraisers. They provide services for senior citizens, the disabled, and other homebound people.

wellness state of human functioning that may be defined as the achievement of one's maximum attainable potential.

Index

Boldface indicates nontext material